Praise for
Cancer: 50 Essential Things to Do

"Patient empowerment at its very best."
—Kenneth H. Cooper, M.D.

"The keys that can open the door for your return to good health."
—O. Carl Simonton, M.D.

"A comprehensive checklist of advice and action steps from a survivor who's been there."
—*Modern Maturity*

The 22 (Non-negotiable) Laws of Wellness

"Read this wonderful book and grow."
—Wayne Dyer, M.D.

"The most comprehensive, easy-to-follow explanation of wellness that I have ever read."
—Edward Taub, M.D., author of *The Wellness Rx*

The Triumphant Patient

"An inspirational classic for people going through illness. A 'gift with a lift' to the human spirit."
—Abigail Van Buren, "Dear Abby"

"Genuine authentic healing hope . . . an absolute inspiration."
—Rev. Robert H. Schuller

Greg Anderson, a survivor of lung cancer, is the best-selling author of six books on health and inspiration, and the founder and chairman of the American Wellness and Cancer Conquerors foundations, national support organizations committed to teaching patients and their families how to cope with cancer.

CANCER

50 ESSENTIAL THINGS TO DO

REVISED AND UPDATED EDITION OF
*50 ESSENTIAL THINGS TO DO
WHEN THE DOCTOR SAYS IT'S CANCER*

GREG ANDERSON

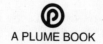

A PLUME BOOK

PLUME
Published by the Penguin Group
Penguin Putnam Inc., 375 Hudson Street, New York, New York 10014, U.S.A.
Penguin Books Ltd, 27 Wrights Lane, London W8 5TZ, England
Penguin Books Australia Ltd, Ringwood, Victoria, Australia
Penguin Books Canada Ltd, 10 Alcorn Avenue, Toronto, Ontario, Canada M4V 3B2
Penguin Books (N.Z.) Ltd, 182–190 Wairau Road, Auckland 10, New Zealand

Penguin Books Ltd, Registered Offices:
Harmondsworth, Middlesex, England

First published by Plume,
a member of Penguin Putnam Inc.
An earlier edition of this book was published by Plume under the title *50 Essential Things to Do When the Doctor Says It's Cancer*.

First Printing, August, 1999
10 9 8 7 6 5 4 3 2 1

  REGISTERED TRADEMARK—MARCA REGISTRADA

Library of Congress Cataloging-in-Publication Data

Anderson, Greg.
    Cancer : 50 essential things to do / Greg Anderson.
        p. cm.
    "Revised edition of 50 Essential things to do when the doctor
says it's cancer."
    ISBN 0-452-28074-5
    1. Cancer—Popular works.   I. Anderson, Greg. 50 things to
do when the doctor says it's cancer.   II. Title.
    RC263 .A617   1999
    616.99'4—dc21   98-53091
                                                          CIP

Printed in the United States of America
Set in Caslon 540
Designed by Leonard Telesca

This book is dedicated to my wife, Linda, and our daughter, Erica.
Your unconditional loving sustains me.

ACKNOWLEDGMENTS

A heartfelt thank-you to all the friends of the Cancer Recovery Foundation of America. I treasure you.

A very special thank-you to the Plume family—especially Audrey LaFehr and Genny Ostertag. I appreciate all you do and all you are.

To all who so generously gave their time, talents, and creativity to this project, please accept my sincere appreciation.

And to all who search these pages for the answers to wellness and to the world, my love.

Contents

FOREWORD

For over twenty-five years, I have been working with an approach to cancer that includes the physical, mental, and spiritual. I have treated thousands of patients with a relatively high rate of recovery, even from so-called "terminal" illness. I have learned a great deal about healing, and I have met some remarkable patients. Greg Anderson is one of them.

This book, *Cancer: 50 Essential Things to Do*, is a testimony to patients taking charge and choosing a stance of hope toward a diagnosis of cancer. Many of you who read this book are undoubtedly in a very difficult situation. Do not despair. Keep your hope alive. Learn from the experience of someone who was given a thirty-days-to-live prognosis. The author has been there. He knows what it's like to deal with the despair of cancer. He also knows what it's like to get well again.

While the road ahead may be difficult, I want you to know that it can be the most rewarding journey you will ever take. Even though the path through cancer requires work and discipline, it is also filled with discoveries that will excite and motivate you. Keep your focus on those joys.

Begin your journey now. Here, in this book, are the keys that can open the door for your return to good health. Take charge. Live this moment. Forgive. Love. You'll then know the power of hope . . . and you will be on the path to getting well again.

—O. Carl Simonton, M.D.
　Founder, Simonton Cancer Center
　Pacific Palisades, California

INTRODUCTION

This revised and updated edition of *Cancer: 50 Essential Things to Do* is written for those people who want to survive the experience of cancer and who are willing to participate actively in the recovery process. The book's goal is twofold: to help you consider the major issues following a cancer diagnosis, and to encourage you to implement a comprehensive recovery plan of your design that has your highest confidence level.

This book is action-oriented, designed to help you put in motion a program that will maximize your opportunity for a complete recovery while maintaining high quality of life. This is not a book to be read and then put away, never to refer to again. Instead, think of using this as your wellness resource guide for the next two years—a reasonable time for recovery. Return to it again and again to get "unstuck" in your cancer journey.

I believe this book has a meaningful message for every person affected by cancer. The strategies are tailor-made for the person with a recent cancer diagnosis. If you have recently been told "It's cancer," you'll find here the information you need to gain control over your fears, analyze your diagnosis, and put in place the most effective integrated treatment program possible. For the newly diagnosed, I recommend following the "50 Essential Things" in order. There is a certain logical progression in their sequence. Following this pattern will prove invaluable and will ensure that you are making the wisest decisions possible.

This book is also written for the person who has been diagnosed with a recurrence of cancer. Recurrence is a frightening event, a time of re-evaluation medically, emotionally, and spiritually. I encourage you to make the "50 Essential Things" the very heart of your entire analysis. Thoughtfully follow the steps. Use this book as your primary guide. A recurrence does not mean certain death. What you do does make a difference! See the "50 Essential Things" as mandatory points of action. Then you'll know you're doing everything possible to contribute to your greater well-being.

This book is also for the "well" cancer patient. That description may seem like a contradiction in terms. It is not. Even those patients who enjoy remission or a complete cure carry with them the lingering fear that cancer may strike again at any time. The "50 Essential Things" will give you the wellness principles you need to assure yourself that you are doing everything possible to retain your good health. Practice the suggestions. They are your best assurance of well-being.

THE WELLNESS AND RECOVERY JOURNAL

Before you begin reading, secure a notebook and a pencil. I want you to create a Wellness and Recovery Journal. I started mine with a single sheet of my daughter's notebook paper and an old three-ring binder, nothing elaborate is required. As you read, questions and insights will come to mind. Write them down. You'll find yourself clipping newspaper and magazine articles about cancer. Put them in your notebook. This is going to become your primary source book, a reference manual for your personal and individualized cancer recovery program. Now, fifteen years after I was told I would die, I have seventeen thick binders that hold a wealth of insights and information important to me. I still add information. My journal also serves as an excellent log that records my cancer recovery journey.

I advise you to do the same. You need the clarity the Wellness and Recovery Journal delivers. Even though a road map to recovery is contained in this book, each person must ultimately chart his or her own course to wellness. Use your Wellness and Recovery Journal to record your unique personal insights. Especially record your questions. Then ask. Ask your doctor, your medical technicians, and other survivors. Nothing is to be assumed. Ask about medical terms that you don't understand. Ask about reasons for tests. Ask about the results of those tests. Ask for success stories. Ask. Ask. Ask. Asking questions gives you significant power. Do not be intimidated by medical personnel or the process. You are the one in charge. Ask! Then record the responses. Come back to them again and again.

Through it all, there is good reason to be filled with hope provided you take an active part in the recovery process. A fighting spirit does make a difference. Let's get started now.

Hershey, Pennsylvania
June 1999

AUTHOR'S NOTE

The ideas in this book are meant to supplement the care and guidance of competent medical professionals. At no time does the author suggest that these steps take the place of conventional medical treatment. Do not attempt a self-diagnosis. Do not embark upon self-treatment of a serious illness without professional help. There are a growing number of informed doctors who will work with their clients to integrate body, mind, and spirit. Find one. Form a healing partnership.

The characters in this book are composites of real people. They are not intended to portray specific individuals.

ESSENTIAL UNDERSTANDING

What's Happening?

A Different Kind of Illness

Cancer is a complex and multi-dimensional process. On the cellular level, cancer is the mutation of genes resulting in the irregular growth of abnormal cells. The operative words here are *irregular* and *abnormal.*

Healthy cells of the body grow in predictable patterns. As they wear out, they are replaced in an orderly manner by just the right number of new healthy cells.

Cancerous cells grow in uncontrolled and unpredictable patterns. Their growth serves no useful biological purpose and often threatens the entire body. The cells themselves are mutant, changed in a way that limits their function.

You have this condition in your body. Your cancer is one of more than 100 types of cancers, each having its own site and distinguishing genetic characteristics.

A second dimension of cancer is its being a symptom of an inefficient immune system. Your understanding of this second point is of vital importance, critical in your decision to do all you can to help yourself get well. Your immune system is the first and most powerful defense your body has against cancer. For years, you have periodically produced mutant cells that were potentially cancerous. In most cases the immune system was there to "clean up" the problems. Now it has ceased doing so in an efficient enough manner to ensure your health.

This book will give specific steps to help you set in place a medical team and an integrated treatment program in which you have confidence, to address the biological portion of the illness. The book will also set out specific physical, psychological, and spiritual action points that will enhance your greater well-being, enrich your life, and ultimately help strengthen your immune system. These action points play an important role in mobilizing your powerful natural healing potential and your self-healing capabilities.

This is the body-mind-spirit connection. It is real and powerful. When used in conjunction with an integrated plan of medical care, this is the combination that creates the optimum environment for your healing. Your medical team will do all it can to remove or control the mutant cells. Your task is to do all you can to enhance your self-healing capacity. Enhancing self-healing is done not so much through medical treatment as it is through your own choices—your physical, emotional, and spiritual lifestyle. In a real sense, I am asking you to enter into "lifestyle therapy," initiating and integrating a comprehensive whole-person recovery effort.

Abundant authoritative, scientifically validated evidence exists that the immune system is profoundly influenced by lifestyle choices. Few people would argue that tobacco use, improper diet, and lack of exercise are obvious deterrents to maximum health. So is mismanaged toxic stress, which fills the body with adrenaline and cortisone derivatives, both known to inhibit immune function.

Something as basic as your emotional reaction to the communication of the cancer diagnosis is a factor. The message "It's cancer" is received with pervasive fear by most people. That fear can paralyze the recipient emotionally and psychologically at a time when intelligent action is required. And a spiritually toxic outlook after a cancer diagnosis can make a difficult situation a living hell. All of these responses have a negative physiological impact on immune function.

After putting your medical team in place, your concentrated efforts must be directed toward your mental, emotional, and spiritual practices if you wish to optimize your chances for recovery. Fail to do so at your own peril. Retaining a medical team without doing all you can to help yourself is like attempting to walk with one stilt. It's possible but the results are frequently disappointing.

The comprehensive integrated whole-person emphasis of this book, and the implementation strategies that flow from this approach, should not cast doubts on the validity of truly scientific medicine. I do not encourage you to go back to the use of folk medicine, though I do have the utmost respect for the old-fashioned family doctor. One problem with scientific medicine is that it is not scientific enough. Evidence supporting a comprehensive approach does exist; in patient after patient we can observe the integrated body-mind-spirit connection at work. But researchers cannot yet measure these obvious effects to their scientific satisfaction, and because the effects cannot be, or have not been, measured in what are called randomized clinical trials, the evidence tends to be dismissed.

I am keenly aware that evidence is not proof. But understand the converse is also true: Lack of evidence does not equal disproof. As we shall see, many widely accepted applications of conventional cancer treatments are based on less-than-complete science.

Modern medicine will become truly scientific only when patients and their medical teams learn to manage the natural forces of the body, mind, and spirit within the context of a program for total well-being. That is what I mean when I encourage you to adopt a comprehensive integrated treatment program.

If you have cancer today, you can't wait for years of medical research to prove these points. This book will provide you with the most up-to-date knowledge available. Integrate these techniques with the best that medicine has to offer. Therein lies optimum success.

Cancer is indeed a different kind of illness that demands a different kind of response. Recovery demands your participation. What you contribute does make a difference. For cancer patients who are determined to conquer this illness, that is very good news indeed.

No Such Thing as Hopeless

You may have been told, "Get your affairs in order," "You have a short time to live," or a favorite of the medical community, "Your illness is terminal." Don't believe it. Refuse to give in to that despair. Only God knows how long a person has to live.

In 1984 I was given a thirty-days-to-live prognosis. It was lung cancer. I'd had one lung removed, but four months later the cancer was back. This time it invaded my lymph system. The surgeon put his hand on my shoulder and said, "Greg, the tiger is out of the cage. Your cancer has come roaring back. I'd give you about thirty days to live."

Part of the reason that surgeon was mistaken is that no health care provider can predict a patient's response to illness. After a couple of days of believing I would die, I made a profound decision. I decided to live!

Please clearly understand what I am saying. By deciding to live I made a decision to do all I could to triumph over the cancer. I determined to live each day I was given to the very best of my ability. I chose not to focus on the despair implicit in the surgeon's words; I would instead adopt a stance of hopefulness. These decisions drastically changed my experience of illness. They resulted not only in better days but many more days as well. I believe such a decision may result in a similar outcome for you.

This message has its critics; it's controversial. More than once, esteemed members of the health care community have publicly accused me of spreading false hope. My answer is simple and direct. I believe there is no such thing as false hope, there is only reasonable hope. Reasonable hope is a medicine worthy of consumption in large doses.

What is clearly false is the pronouncement that sets a limit on the amount of time a cancer patient may have left to live. That's "false hopelessness." It is false because no human being knows how long anyone has left to live. To prognosticate in such a manner is not only unprofessional, it is unethical. Healers instill hope. They do not schedule death.

So decide to live! Embrace hope. Hope heals. It is a decision that always leads to better days and perhaps more of them as well.

I deeply empathize with you and your health crisis. I have been there. I have been torn by the same emotions that now rip at you. I can identify with your fear and uncertainty. It is the most frightening time of your life.

Before you lie two paths. One is marked by passiveness and despair; the other by the guideposts of active involvement and hope. You have a choice; you can always choose hope. If you have been told that your time is limited, believe that life can still be a fulfilling adventure. Choose to live life to the very fullest. Focus on that potential rather than the problem. Discover that every day is a good and perfect gift in spite of the circumstances of illness. In that intentional choice lie the seeds of your healing. Water the seeds, not the weeds.

Without question, you can improve your potential for survival. What you do does make a significant difference. There is no such thing as a hopeless situation.

Promise yourself, promise me, that you will always choose and act on hope.

A
ROAD
MAP TO
RECOVERY

LEARNING FROM THE TRUE EXPERTS

After my surgeon told me I had 30 days to live, I was stunned. One moment I was in tears, the next I was enraged. I thought it was all a mistake; I was convinced my tests had been confused with another patient's. I was filled with fear and self-pity. One afternoon I yelled out in anger, "Oh God, what can I do?"

That question was the right query. And it was answered. No, God didn't part the clouds and speak; I remain a committed skeptic regarding such claims. But figuratively, the clouds were parted and God did communicate. It was a non-verbal communication. I had the distinct impression that my task was to search for survivors. I became aware that I needed to find people who were "supposed" to die but had lived. And once I found them, I was to learn from their experience.

To date, I have interviewed and received surveys from more than 15,000 survivors of "terminal" illness. These are the people who have been told the equivalent of "Get your affairs in order.

You are about to die." They are the brave patients who, at one time, had no hope, the people whom the medical community wrote off. But these same people lived!

These inspiring individuals, who possess no more courage or ability than you or I, teach some powerful lessons from which we can learn. These ideas and practices have worked successfully for me and for tens of thousands of other cancer patients. I believe the lessons can also be pivotal in your life and your health.

After I conducted over 500 interviews, it became clear there were similar patterns to most of the individual outcomes. For example, the vast majority of survivors do not believe they recovered their health by chance. The triumphant patients believe they worked for their wellness, earning it on a daily basis. Neither do most survivors credit their doctors alone, or even primarily, for their recovery. Instead, the exceptional patients focus on personally mobilizing body, mind, and spirit in their quest for high-level wellness.

Pattern after pattern emerged from the survivor interviews. In 1988 I first summarized the strategies and combined them into a simple plan that anyone could understand and put to use. The plan has since been refined by thousands of additional interviews and experiences. Today, through the Cancer Recovery Foundation of America's Cancer Recovery Program, thousands of cancer patients have used these principles as a road map, a strategic plan, to enhance their health and enrich their lives.

THE EIGHT STRATEGIES

Before we come to the "50 Essential Things," I'd like to review the eight basic strategies that cancer survivors have in common. The following emerged from the survivor interviews.

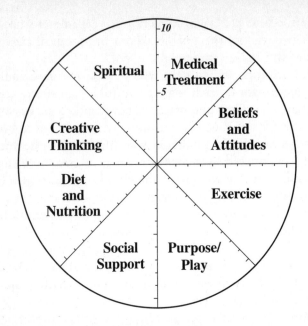

Rate Yourself: After reading and studying each of the eight strategies, return to this diagram and give yourself a rating for each category. 10=highest, 1=lowest. What does this tell you about your wellness and about your cancer journey? Take a break from your reading and consider the implications of this analysis.

Strategy #1: Medical Treatment

Over 96 percent of cancer survivors start and complete a treatment program grounded in conventional medical care. Surgery, radiation therapy, chemotherapy, hormonal therapy, and immunotherapy—often in combination—are the treatments of choice.

This much is clear: The overwhelming majority of cancer survivors do undergo conventional medical treatment. This is a critically important message.

I was both surprised and encouraged by this. I thought I might find survivors using nontraditional methods like exotic diets and "secret" potions. Yes, there were some who subscribed to such alternative approaches. But more than 96 out of 100 patients adopted a treatment plan based on recognized conventional Western medical protocols.

However, there are two extremely important footnotes to this fact. First, survivors demand hard evidence that the suggested treatments are effective, and second, survivors do not stop with conventional medical treatments.

As you study the "50 Essential Things," you'll see how survivors literally take charge of the management of their entire medical program: They choose doctors in whom they have confidence; they consent only to treatment programs about which they have convictions; and survivors aggressively integrate complementary and alternative treatment approaches.

Nutritional programs are common. So, too, is psychospiritual work. Survivors are active patients, involved with each decision, making certain that they are fully informed and understand each recovery component. Taking charge of one's medical treatment program, and the perception of control that follows, is a prominent theme in cancer survivorship.

Strategy #2: Beliefs and Attitudes

Do beliefs and attitudes heal? Survivors believe so. Cancer survivors choose beliefs and attitudes about their illness, as well as their potential for wellness, that empower. The most fundamental and empowering belief is that cancer does not equate with death.

It is sad but true that much of the world still considers cancer and death to be synonymous, but that is not so among survivors.

However, the majority of survivors are not "be-positive-against-all-evidence" thinkers. They have a refreshing sense of skepticism about "just-think-positive" solutions. Survivors tend to be tough-minded realists, people who clearly understand what cancer may mean. Very few survivors have an attitude that says, "No problem. I'm fine. Everything's going to be all right." That's clearly denial.

Instead, survivors recognize this truth—cancer may or may not mean death. This intellectual stance carries a vastly different outlook from either the super-positive or hopelessly negative beliefs and attitudes. Survivors believe, "Yes, I may die. But I also may live. And I am going to invest my time, whatever the length, in living the best way I know." Survival often follows this pronouncement.

Survivors also tend to hold unique beliefs about their medical treatment. They challenge the conventional thinking about treatment and potential side effects. They choose to conceive of their treatment as highly effective, believing that they will have minimal and manageable side effects. The "50 Essential Things" will help you understand and apply these key beliefs and attitudes in your own treatment program.

You probably will not be surprised to learn that survivors hold another key belief about their role in illness recovery. They believe their active personal involvement is absolutely essential to the recovery process. Survivors have a healthy "work ethic." They believe wellness is no accident, that it requires effort, and that it is their personal responsibility to make getting well the number one priority in their lives. For the moment, getting well takes precedence over everything. Survivors hold firmly to the belief that what they personally contribute to recovery makes a significant difference.

"Cancer does not equate with death. Treatment is effective. I have a significant role to play." These powerful foundational beliefs and attitudes help focus the efforts of survivors. Many survivors feel these positive beliefs and attitudes themselves have a biochemical reality that enhances healing; a growing body of credible scientific evidence supports this position. You'll recognize these beliefs and attitudes throughout the "50 Essential Things."

Strategy #3: Exercise

Cancer survivors believe strongly in the importance of exercise, and they act on that belief. Nearly nine out of every ten people I interviewed emphasized the need for regular physical activity. There were swimmers, bikers, and lots of walkers. Most surprising were those patients who started exercise programs even while they were confined to hospital beds or in wheelchairs or were otherwise physically limited. They would do full-body stretches in bed, lift weights from chairs, and do everything possible to honor their physical needs. It was inspiring to hear the stories.

Before my cancer diagnosis, I did not exercise. Other than an occasional game of tennis or a monthly golf outing, I was a sedentary person. I came face-to-face with my own exercise attitudes and habits early in my recovery journey. Exercise ranked second only to developing a belief that recovery was possible, in starting me on the path to well-being.

It was not easy. I lay weak, emaciated, and sedated in our guest bedroom. Even with medication, I felt the pain. I had no energy. But I wanted to live. And I was willing to do the work required for healing.

I started the telephone interviews searching for survivors. I repeatedly heard the admonition to exercise. Initially, I resisted and I argued for my limits. "I'm confined to bed. I'm weak. I'm in pain. How could I ever exercise?"

Finally, convinced that it might be possible to exercise through the pain and that I would benefit from it, I began with chair exercises. I would do the backstroke, the windmill motions, with my arms. Ten clockwise, ten counterclockwise, just until I felt an increase in energy. In a few days I added some leg lifts, still from a seated position. At first, my total exercise time was five minutes, perhaps less. Then I extended it to twice a day. Next I increased each session 10 minutes.

As I gained strength, I added a short walking routine, first for just a few minutes, later to 10, 15, then 20 minutes. I made certain I followed the increase-in-energy guidelines you'll find in the forthcoming pages. Soon I understood firsthand the profound effect of what other survivors told me: "Take charge of your body. Command your body to move."

Exercise is a key recovery strategy, more powerful than I ever imagined. I predict you will come to see that exercise which you enjoy is an important part of your own recovery regimen.

Strategy #4: Purpose/Play Balance

Purpose involves survivors perceiving that they are needed, that their life has special and unique meaning. Many are energized by an inner, even transcendent, life mission. Survivors balance this profound idea of life purpose with a lighter, more playful attitude of fun for fun's sake, an outlook that creates joy. These seemingly contradictory positions are major recurring themes among the community of cancer survivors.

A sense of purpose is powerful. Survivors first cultivate mission. The feeling of being needed and wanted expresses itself in many ways. Service to others is the consistent theme. Family is a reason: "They couldn't get along without me." Important accomplishments or life milestones also enrich the life purpose for many survivors: "I determined I was going to participate in my daughter's wedding." "I'm going to live to see my grandchild born."

An important note is that most survivors are able to separate being needed from being unduly depended upon. Few are rescuers or feel forced to serve. Instead, survivors feel that they are privileged to be able to help others in meaningful ways. In helping others, they help themselves, thus reinforcing the perception that they are wanted and needed. Survivors balance this deep sense of purpose with play. It's more than fun; it's something much deeper, a cultivation of joy. Hobbies engage this extraordinary group of people. I am struck by the large number who enjoy gardening, both flowers and vegetables. Male, female, city or rural, it doesn't seem to make much difference. Many survivors express deep satisfaction in seeing their efforts produce new life. I sense that the growing plants serve as a metaphor for their own journeys to a new and better life resulting from the cancer experience.

Strategy #5: Social Support

Cancer survivors invest more time and emotional energy in relationships that nurture them and invest less in those that are toxic. While this may seem like a benign practice, it has some surprising health implications that survivors believe are central to their success.

Loving relationships with friends, relatives, lovers, spouses, children, employers, coworkers, and employees—or the lack of these relationships—build us up or tear us down. Survivors become "relationship sensitive," examining, perhaps for the first time in their lives, how they get along with other people. It is common for survivors to put difficult relationships "on hold," especially during the medical treatment process. This doesn't mean survivors automatically exile "toxic" people from their lives for all time. But it certainly signals a reduced emotional and spiritual investment in those relationships.

Cancer tends to give patients permission to examine a wide variety of their life choices, including their entire social support system. Changes often follow. Much of the actual work of getting well again takes place within the social support arena. New and important research is giving credibility to the relationship between positive social support and health.

Social support extends to support groups. Cancer survivors know the importance of mutual aid, having practiced it long before support groups became fashionable and prior to research pointing to the measurable benefits of participation. Today the proliferation of cancer support groups puts this service within reach for any person who desires to attend. Authoritative research shows survival rates doubled for support group participants when compared with non-joiners. Survivors make support groups and positive social support a central part of their recovery process.

Strategy #6: Diet and Nutrition

The majority of cancer survivors report making significant dietary changes. There is wide recognition of the important contribution diet makes to recovery and to ongoing health. However, there is anything but universal agreement on exactly what those specific changes should be.

One thing we can say with certainty, "Survivors eat with awareness." They raise their nutritional IQ and develop a greater understanding of the nutrients contained in their food selections. Survivors also feed themselves less for emotional and psychological reasons, concentrating instead on delivering premium nutrients to the body. They embrace foods that are less processed. There is a documented shift to a more vegetarian approach. Fresh fruits, fresh vegetables, and whole grains are the new foods of choice. A marked decrease in all meat, particularly red meat, is widely held to be beneficial.

While vitamin, mineral, and herbal supplementation is widely practiced among survivors, there exists a lack of consensus in actual practices. Some survivors use many supplements; others settle for a daily multiple vitamin.

One survivor consensus I can report on in the arena of diet and nutrition is that of attitude. While the specific nutritional practices vary, survivors do agree on one thing. They have an excited belief that nutrition is another thing they get to focus on to recover their health. Survivors perceive diet as another point of personal control. It's an area in which they can take charge in the sometimes out-of-control cancer experience.

Strategy #7: Creative Thinking

Survivors mobilize the mind to heal. Affirmations, meditation, and imagery are widely employed within the context of a comprehensive treatment program. Survivors use meditative techniques to reduce the symptoms of illness, manage the side effects of treatment, and improve emotional well-being.

Our culture tells us that positive feelings are desirable and negative feelings are not. Survivors have a more realistic way of viewing emotions. They tend to accept whatever emotions they have, be they positive or negative. Survivors are typically realists who recognize that the cancer journey has tremendous emotional hills and valleys. So they simply accept the emotions that accompany these roller coaster feelings.

But grasp this key emotional insight: Survivors do not become stuck in any single emotion. They do not cling to fear or anger; they are able to recognize negative feelings and choose more empowering emotions. It's creative thinking at its best.

I am struck by how many survivors use affirmations in the management of their emotions. As an example, survivors tend to focus on living in the present moment. They use affirmations, a simple phrase or verse, to gain emotional comfort and control rather than allowing runaway thoughts and feelings to rule their lives.

The "50 Essential Things" will detail several creative thinking options, support them with credible up-to-date research, and help you implement them in your own recovery program. For survivors, the mind is another powerful resource to mobilize in the getting-well journey.

Strategy #8: Spirituality

Survivors embrace a more spiritual perspective. They view life differently than prior to their brush with death. While some cancer patients focus on a body that may be riddled with disease or mourn over dreams that are hopelessly derailed, survivors tend to see the high value of what is simple and readily available in spite of their cancer.

To call spirituality a "strategy" is inadequate; "spiritual transformation" is a more accurate description. Thousands of survivors demonstrate entirely new spirit; they become new people.

This more spiritual personal demeanor is not necessarily an issue of religion—many survivors reject traditional religious practices. No single doctrine or creed brings pre-packaged answers to all. Nor does this more universal spirituality simply consist of sweet platitudes. For many, it is a radical but serene response to recovery and to life. It's discovering the divinity within; experiencing inner peace. For thousands of cancer survivors, this is the apex of the healing journey.

IMPLEMENTATION INTELLIGENCE

Each of the eight strategies is important, but they are not always equal. For example, the timing varies: At initial diagnosis, nearly all the emphasis may be placed on medical treatment. This is appropriate. After the treatment program is in place, survivors may then place more emphasis on beliefs and attitudes or diet and nutrition. Only later may they begin the work of social support or focus on another principle.

Each survivor creates his or her own specific recovery plan within the structure of these eight strategies. One principle takes priority at the appropriate time. Seldom do survivors make simultaneous wholesale changes in all eight areas. Those who attempt to change too much too quickly often meet with temporary defeat and have to start again.

Each strategy has its important place in the recovery program of most cancer patients. Even though there is a difference in timing, many survivors note, in retrospect, that resolving a relationship problem may have been just as important in their recovery as medical treatment! The positive signals that proper diet and regular exercise give to the body are so strong that many survivors rate diet and exercise on a par with, or even above, the contribution of radiation or chemotherapy.

Nearly all survivors agree it is the balance, the comprehensive integrated approach that includes, but does not stop at, conventional medicine, that makes recovery possible.

In the final analysis, most survivors feel they earn their return to health. But this is not viewed as some extraordinary event. Survivors speak more about aligning themselves with the body's immense natural power to heal itself. Indeed, survivors come to recognize that health and healing spring from within. They simply had to release them.

Let's summarize to this point. The integration of these eight strategies create the framework for cancer patients to follow in the recovery process:

Medical Treatment   Social Support
Beliefs and Attitudes   Diet and Nutrition
Exercise   Creative Thinking
Purpose/Play Balance   Spirituality

This strategic plan is the context in which the "50 Essential Things" are implemented. It's your map. Consult it often.

THE
50
ESSENTIAL
THINGS
TO DO

DETERMINING YOUR TREATMENT PROGRAM

Your number one priority following a cancer diagnosis is to put in place the best integrated medical treatment program you can possibly obtain. But this is not as simple as going to one doctor and saying, "Treat me."

The decisions you make authorizing your conventional cancer treatment program are some of the most important you will make in your entire life. Begin the journey through cancer by following this course of action that has proven highly effective for thousands of cancer survivors.

#1

STOP
"AWFULIZING"

You've been told "It's cancer." I have deep compassion for you. I fully appreciate your feelings. I've been there, too.

First, you're in shock, and filled with fear. The next moment you're angry but not quite certain at what or whom. Then comes the thoughts of "How did this happen? Why me?" Even the guilt starts to creep in, "Did I bring this on myself?" Plus, all the questions have started to rush through your mind: "Will I die?" "How long do I have?" "What will happen to my family?" and on and on and on. Your mind is overwhelmed at times.

Be calm. Try not to panic. I know that this is easier said than done, but be aware that panic will only inhibit rational and positive action.

Cancer is a serious illness but it is not necessarily fatal. You do have the luxury of some time. Unlike a severed artery, cancer does not require you to do something this very instant. A hurried response, based in the emotions of fear and panic, is neither required nor preferred. In fact, a hurried response may be harmful. Don't take that as a license for inaction, however.

Stop and examine your frenzied thoughts for just a moment. It is at the beginning stages of this journey that clear decision-making will be most important. With these early decisions, you will ensure that your illness is properly treated. Panic acts only to your detriment.

Panic is a mental phenomenon, a response to our thoughts about cancer being frightful and overpowering. The process can accurately be labeled as "awfulizing." Isn't that an apt description? When we awfulize, we take our current situation to its worst possible conclusion.

If we will observe our emotions objectively for just a moment, we will see something different from initial appearances. The intense panic that virtually every cancer patient experiences is actually the mind projecting its fears about the unknown future. Think about it, and understand this truth: Panic is caused by an assumption. It is not based on material fact.

We are not made up of just our fears. Our fears do not necessarily determine our future. This is a profound healing insight.

What to do when you start to feel anxious emotions arising inside? Try to witness them. Just observe. You may want to give those emotions an image. View them, and yourself, in your mind's eye. Instead of putting yourself in the role of a victim who is hopelessly caught in a web of panic and despair, become the observer. By not engaging the mind in battle, by simply watching the emotions and letting go, your panic will soon subside.

Then imagine yourself as an effective problem solver. Give yourself an image of a competent and confident person who is about to make some very important choices. Clear decision-making can and will be yours.

An Important Thing You Can Do

Sit down. Take a deep breath. Say out loud, "Cancer does not mean death." Observe your emotions. Detach by separating who you are as a person from the emotional panic you may be feeling. You are not uncontrolled panic even though you may be experiencing panic. Understand that difference. Then immediately read and act on the next two steps in this book.

#2

TAKE
CHARGE

Who is the most important person on our cancer recovery team? Some people believe it is their surgeon. Others believe it is their oncologist. Some choose the medical technicians, others the nurse, and still others choose their spouse.

But the most important person on your wellness team is you! You are the one who is ill. It is you who must work to get well again. You are the character of central importance. You are in charge.

Too often patients surrender leadership. Elizabeth, a 38-year-old housewife, was diagnosed with metastatic breast cancer. Her treatment was not progressing as expected, and the side effects depleted her. It all left Elizabeth understandably discouraged. Her doctor kept assuring her, "We're doing all we can. Trust me."

Following an especially difficult week, Elizabeth asked herself, "Do I accept the course of this treatment or do I try something new?" She called and made an appointment at a Clinical Cancer Center that was a four-hour drive from her home. Doctors there recommended a different treatment program that Elizabeth took back to her home doctor for implementation. "Personally taking charge was my turning point," explained a healthy Elizabeth four years after her bold and assertive decision.

Survivors take charge. View yourself as the manager of a baseball team, or whatever organizational analogy you like. This is your cancer recovery team. The team's mission is to get you well again. You'll want a strong starting pitcher; many times that is the oncologist. And you'll need many other team members: a catcher, infielders, outfielders. Equate these with specialists. You, the manager, choose the team that is on the field at any given moment.

Taking charge is a significant step for many patients. Traditionally, consumers play a passive role in the health care system, going along with virtually whatever doctors and allied health care professionals recommend. We're encouraged to consent to rather than challenge recommendations. This passive attitude does not serve you well. Decide to take charge now!

An Important Thing You Can Do

Evaluate your team. Who are the players? Who is managing this team? Is it a one-person show, when many more people could be helping? Are the team members working for you or do some seem to be working against you? One woman remarked, "Every time I go to the doctor, I feel like I am in enemy territory." If you feel that way, it may be a signal that you need to make a substitution. Remember: You are the person in charge!

#3

Ask Your Doctor These Questions

It is critically important for you to clearly understand your diagnosis and the proposed treatment. The doctor who diagnosed you should answer the following questions. Record the answers:

1. Precisely what type of cancer do I have?_____
2. Has the cancer spread beyond the primary site? If so, where?

_____

3. What tests did you use to determine this diagnosis?

_____

4. Is there any indication that a second pathology report is needed?

_____

5. Are you recommending additional tests? What are you looking for with each test?

_____

_____

6. How certain are you that the tests and the resulting diagnosis are accurate?

_____

7. What are my treatment options? Which one(s) do you recommend? (Record these recommendations in precise detail.)

_____

_____

8. Will you obtain and review with me the treatment information on my type and stage of cancer from the National Cancer Institute's Physicians Data Query (PDQ) program?

_____

9. Whom would you recommend for a second opinion?

_____

10. Are you a board-certified oncologist?

_____

As a cancer patient you are a consumer. The decision process regarding who will prescribe and administer your treatment is not that much different from any other major purchase decision. But the consequences of your decisions are radically different from those involved in buying an automobile, for example. You have the right, even the responsibility, to ask questions of your doctor just as you would with any consumer purchase. Evaluate those answers more closely than any major purchase you have ever made. Your options and choices for the best treatment will then become clear.

Cancer survivors are consumer activists. They ask. Become an activist!

An Important Thing You Can Do

Obtain answers to the preceding questions today! Record the answers in your Wellness and Recovery Journal. Ask them once again at the time you obtain your second opinion.

#4

GET A
SECOND
OPINION

Obtain a second opinion from a board-certified oncologist, a cancer specialist. This is a critically important step that is not to be overlooked. If at all possible, the second opinion should be completed prior to starting any treatment program.

Whom you consult is also critically important. The second opinion should come from an independent oncologist who is not in a working partnership, formal or informal, with the doctor who made the initial diagnosis. If possible, the second opinion should be given by an oncologist who is in a different medical group from the first. Many people travel to major cancer centers to obtain them. Second opinion consultations are that important.

Do not be fearful that a request for a second opinion might alienate your doctor. Second opinion consultations are standard procedure; your doctor makes such referrals every day. Ask the doctor, or a member of the staff, who made the initial diagnosis for a complete transcript of your medical records. Then take the records with you, or have them sent ahead. I prefer to personally hand the records to the consulting staff. It eliminates the chance of lost pages and delays.

The cost of obtaining second opinions is reimbursed by virtually all insurance programs. Even if you're not covered, get a second opinion. Don't let cost stand in the way of obtaining some of the most important information of your life.

"I had a second opinion all right," explained Katherine, a 55-year-old insurance office manager and grandmother, describing her experience with breast cancer. "The second opinion came from another surgeon who shared offices with the first. They both said that a radical [mastectomy] was the way to go. And to this day I wonder if I would have been better off with a lumpectomy and radiation."

Katherine's second opinion experience could have been improved in two ways. First, she would have been better served by consulting with an oncologist. These specialists diagnose and treat cancer every working day. They can be expected to have the most up-to-date information on treatment options for each type and stage of cancer. Both surgeons Katherine consulted were general surgeons who dealt with a variety of illnesses, not just cancer.

Second, Katherine would have been better served by consulting with a second opinion doctor not associated with the first. Her surgeons were located in the same building and just down the hall from her family doctor.

These associations are a little discussed but potentially important issue to patients. Doctors who are friends, office mates, business associates, or in a junior position within a medical practice may find it difficult to challenge the diagnoses or recommended treatment programs of associates. All sorts of relationships exist that may influence decisions. "We were in the middle of renegotiating the lease," said Robert, a young oncologist who rented office space from another oncologist. "We were meeting that very afternoon to discuss rents. I didn't want to offend my landlord when he sent me a patient for a second opinion consultation. So I just agreed with his treatment recommendations."

That experience may seem improbable, but the story is unfortunately true. The best safeguard is to seek a second opinion from a board-certified oncologist who is affiliated with a different practice, a different hospital, perhaps even lives in a different city than the doctor making the initial diagnosis.

One of the very best places to get a second opinion is from a National Cancer Institute-designated Comprehensive Cancer Center. If those centers are simply too far away from your home, contact the Cancer Information Service, referred to in the next step, to find alternatives nearer you.

It puzzles me why so many cancer patients are fearful of asking for a second opinion. When I have inquired, the typical response is, "No one told me to ask," or, "I don't want to offend my doctor."

Obtaining a second opinion in no way implies that the initial diagnosis is incorrect or that the suggested treatment is inappropriate. On a subject as important as this, you simply deserve to have the benefit of more than one person's thinking. Your second opinion search also puts you in touch with other doctors, giving you options and helping you decide which medical team will actually administer your treatment program.

John was a 62-year-old accountant diagnosed with colon cancer. His primary care doctor suggested John consult with a surgeon. The day John's second set of test results came back from the lab, the surgeon called John, confirmed the initial diagnosis, and said, "I've scheduled you for surgery. Be at the hospital by six-thirty tomorrow morning." Fortunately, John had the courage to say "slow down" and went about obtaining another second opinion consultation from a board-certified oncologist.

The second opinion oncologist independently confirmed the initial diagnosis. In fact, he also recommended surgery, just as John was initially advised. John returned to his surgeon only to be greeted with sarcasm: "I told you so. What's the matter? Didn't you trust me?" John walked out of that doctor's office, found another surgeon, and today is in excellent health. The lessons: Second opinions are critical. And, you do not have to accept medical arrogance.

An Important Thing You Can Do

Make your appointment for a second opinion today. This is one of the most important things you can do. *Do not overlook this step*. Act now! Pick up the phone. Make the appointment.

#5

MAKE AN
IMPORTANT
INQUIRY

You have several important resources to assist you in understanding your physical diagnosis and evaluating conventional treatment options. They are just a phone call or a mouse click away and can link you to information vital to your informed decision-making.

**National Cancer Institute's Cancer Information Service (CIS)
Phone: (800) 4CANCER [422-6237]; web site:
cancernet.nci.nih.gov**

CIS is designed to give you up-to-date, accurate, and understandable information and facts about your type of cancer. Staff consultants give advice on diagnoses, treatment options, treatment guidelines, research news, and other important developments. Have them send you information on your specific type of cancer, the most important information being the state-of-the-art treatment options for your type and stage.

CIS also provides access to PDQ (Physicians Data Query), the largest resource base on conventional cancer treatments. Ask your doctor to review this information with you.

CIS maintains data on centers where investigators are testing experimental therapies. These investigational protocols may be right for you but are generally considered only after conventional treatments have proven unsatisfactory.

American Cancer Society
Phone: (800) 227-2345; web site: www.cancer.org

Staff health consultants answer questions, mail brochures, and make referrals to local medical centers. This web site is the best for understandable information on diagnoses and conventional treatment. The American Cancer Society web site also has numerous links to related web pages.

Cancer Recovery Foundation of America
Phone: (800) 238-6479; web site: www.wellness.net

The best balance between authoritative and user-friendly information comparing conventional, complementary, and alternative treatments. This site rates treatment options by documented outcomes. Staff volunteers also offer counseling that specializes in integrating body, mind, and spirit.

An Important Thing You Can do

Contact the National Cancer Institute, the American Cancer Society, and/or the Cancer Recovery Foundation of America today. Become informed. Hold yourself accountable, at the least, for having an intelligent working knowledge of the type and stage of your cancer diagnosis. And become knowledgeable on the preferred choices in conventional, complementary, and alternative treatments. Record your findings in your Wellness and Recovery Journal.

#6

RETHINK
THE
STATISTICS

As you conduct the research into your conventional, complementary, and alternative treatment options, you will invariably discover cancer recovery statistics that detail cancer incidence, mortality, and five-year survival rates. Do not let these statistics paralyze you. Your response to them is critical.

Statistics measure populations. They can be interpreted in a great many ways. But statistics do not determine any individual case, including yours.

Just after my second surgery, I received a booklet filled with numerical tables, statistics, and graphs on all types of cancers. Of course I felt compelled to read all the information on lung cancer. The numbers on metastatic lung cancer were not promising. As I reflected on what I read, I felt frightened, depressed, and filled with despair, certain of my fast-approaching death.

Several days later I looked again at those statistics and realized that many people do survive. "What did they do?" I wondered. "How can I learn from them?"

No matter how difficult your situation, you must realize that there is no type of cancer that does not have some rate of survival. This is a significant fact, and it is cause for reasonable hope. The question now becomes, "What can I do to maximize my chances of getting on the right side of these statistics?"

With this book you have already begun to tap into the answers.

An Important Thing You Can Do

Interpret statistics as indications of progress. Determine to act with the conviction that hope is your greatest ally and that you will be counted among the "survivor statistics."

#7

UNDERSTAND YOUR CONVENTIONAL TREATMENT OPTIONS

In addition to the information you generate from your own research, you should expect your oncologist to carefully explain which types of conventional treatment are recommended for your type and stage of cancer. The options will typically fall into one or a combination of three primary treatment modalities:

- Surgery: removal of the tumor by operating on it
- Radiation: exposure to x-rays or radium
- Chemotherapy: the use of cytotoxic chemicals

Surgery is the most frequently employed cancer treatment. It is best used when the cancer is small and has not moved to other parts of the body. Radiation therapy is employed in approximately one-half of all cancer cases. It is often used in combination with other treatment options, for example either before or after surgery. Chemotherapy is most often used when the cancer has spread or when the diagnosis is a systemic-type cancer. It is often used in combination with radiation therapy and surgery to control tumor growth.

Three other types of conventional medical treatment modalities are:

- Hormonal: employs or manipulates bodily hormones
- Immunotherapy: enhancing the body's own immune function
- Investigative: experimental programs

Hormonal treatment is used in cancers that depend on hormones for their growth. Hormones are either removed, added, or their production is blocked through drugs or surgery that removes the hormone-producing gland. Immunotherapies include the cytokines like the family of interleukins and interferons, and are an attempt to boost or restore the body's natural defense system. Many people believe immunotherapies will soon comprise a fourth widely accepted treatment modality. At this writing, their scientific efficacy is yet to be established. Investigative protocols are experimental. They are typically the last choice.

As you evaluate your conventional treatment options, I ask you to consider some of my personal observations from a decade and a half of helping patients make informed choices:

1. While surgery is the most common form of conventional treatment, dozens of types of cancer diagnosis do not indicate surgery. Many patients panic when they are told their cancer is "inoperable." If you have been told that your cancer is inoperable, do not despair. Recognize that inoperable does not equate with incurable!

2. If your oncologist suggests surgery, and you concur, the decision as to who actually performs the procedure is yours. Your choice of surgeons is important. You're more likely to get a well-qualified surgeon if you choose one who is a fellow of the American College of Surgeons and who is also board-certified in his or her field. Only about half of practicing surgeons are board-certified, so be sure to ask.

Special note to premenopausal breast cancer patients:

You typically have some flexibility on the timing of your surgery. Scientific evidence is mounting that fewer breast cancer recurrences are reported among women who choose to have their surgery during the luteal phase of the menstrual cycle, i.e., 14–30 days following the onset of menstruation. Except for one Canadian study which suggested Day 8 to be the optimal time, research shows surgery performed in the latter half of the menstrual cycle results in the fewest recurrences. Ask your surgeon for the most up-to-date research information prior to scheduling. You may have to assert yourself here; most surgeries are scheduled at the convenience of the surgeon and/or the hospital.

3. Thoroughly understand chemotherapy. Before you say yes to chemotherapy, ask to see proof, such as scientific papers and reports, on the effectiveness of the treatment being offered. Examine the hard evidence that the suggested chemotherapy protocol actually *cures, extends life, or improves quality of life.* Those are the three "outcomes" against which you must measure all treatments—conventional, experimental, complementary, and alternative.

If your clinician uses the terms "response" or "tumor response" or "reduce the tumor burden," these represent different standards. These terms mean shrinkage and a corresponding reduction in the immune-suppressive effect the tumor has. None of these terms are synonymous with a cure, which actually requires that your body fight the cancer on a cellular level and that your immune system maintain a disease-free state. To maximize your opportunity for such a response, I encourage you to follow as many of the health-enhancing, life-enriching principles in this book as possible.

Study the chemotherapy treatment option in depth. Do your own research. Ask about both short-term and long-term side effects. Request the names and phone numbers of long-term survivors who were treated with similar regimens. Ask for their experience and analysis. Know exactly what you can expect—and not expect—this treatment option to accomplish. Once you possess that information, you are in a position to make a truly informed decision. (See Appendix A, page 172, for a more detailed discussion of chemotherapy options.)

4. The administration of chemotherapy is not an exact science. Ask your oncologist about chemotherapy sensitivity (in vitro) testing. Here, samples of your tissue are chemically analyzed in laboratory tests to determine interaction with different agents. In about a week, your oncologist will receive a report establishing which drugs are not likely to work as well as the most active agents. The net effect is a personalized treatment program optimized before you begin. Do not panic if there are changes in the treatment program. It is common to try different chemotherapy drugs as well as different combinations. These changes are the oncologist's attempt to improve the effectiveness of the treatment.

5. Chemotherapy may be in pill form, and be taken by mouth, or it may be in liquid form and injected into a muscle or, most commonly, given through a vein. The drugs may be administered in a daily, weekly, or monthly program for periods ranging from a few months to a lifetime in a few cases. Side effects, once the fear of all patients, are now being more effectively controlled and vary widely from individual to individual. Refer in this book to #36, "Minimize Treatment Side Effects," for helpful things you can do to control uncomfortable side effects.

6. Radiation therapy is most often administered by means of an external beam machine, though internal radiation is becoming more common. Here, radioactive material is surgically implanted into or on the area to be treated. This procedure requires precision. You will maximize your opportunity for receiving excellent care if you choose a physician who is certified by the American Board of Radiology. Ask.

All cancers are treatable. Even in cases where the cancer is advanced, experimental investigative programs are available. If your cancer is not responding to conventional treatment, ask about hormonal treatment and biological response modifiers. Especially consider the many complementary and alternative programs described in this book. You are entitled to understand the full range of treatments available. From that understanding, you will have the knowledge and power to make the most intelligent treatment decisions.

Once again, conventional treatment has its important place. In interviews with thousands of cancer survivors, over 96 percent stated they initiated a course of conventional therapy. It is a myth that cancer survivors turn exclusively to alternative, nontraditional cancer treatments in large numbers. In the late 1980s, a Food and Drug Administration study estimated that 40 percent of cancer patients use unconventional treatments. That may be true; in fact, I believe the number may now be much higher, perhaps 60 percent. But survivors do not give up the traditional treatments. They integrate complementary and alternative practices into a comprehensive recovery program. That is what the guidance in this book is all about.

A final thought on conventional treatment options:

Please clearly understand this point: The vast majority of survivors select a conventional program using surgery, chemotherapy, or radiation, often in combination, as the foundation of their treatment. Survivors then supplement this conventional approach with many of the ideas presented in this book. I recommend you implement a conventional medical treatment program based on your own research and your own strong belief. However, I also believe your treatment is not complete until you initiate a comprehensive and integrated recovery program. Given our current levels of understanding, this integration represents your very best opportunity for surviving cancer.

An Important Thing You Can Do

Ask your oncologist to explain the specific treatment options available to you in the areas of surgery, radiation, and chemotherapy. Ask also about hormonal, immunotherapy, and investigative programs. Ask for his or her recommendation. Record this information in your Wellness and Recovery Journal. *Do not* give your approval for treatment just yet. First, more work remains to be completed.

#8

GAUGE YOUR CONFIDENCE IN YOUR MEDICAL TEAM

Few patients have any objective way to judge whether their surgeons, oncologists, or other medical professionals have technical competence. We can consider our medical team's education and professional certifications, and the experiences of other patients. But few of us can evaluate, with technical accuracy, whether a particular doctor will be able to address our specific case with success. We can, however, make subjective assessments, the kind of judgments that can be enormously important in any recovery journey. We can intuitively gauge our confidence level.

Ann, a highly successful insurance executive, was diagnosed with ovarian cancer. By the time it was discovered, the metastasis was significant and the prognosis poor. Ann interviewed seven different oncologists. She went to them with her pathology report and diagnosis in hand and simply asked, "Assuming this diagnosis is correct, what would you have me do?"

The answers she received were actually fairly predictable and consistent. That was reassuring. But what was more comforting was one oncologist's interpersonal skills. He listened. He asked questions to determine Ann's confidence in a procedure. Based on Ann's answers, and her confidence level, he offered his recommendations. Ann chose this doctor.

Ann's analysis was based not so much on any objective measures of technical competence but on her intuition, her belief in a person and the recommended program. She followed that intuition.

I believe you can trust your intuition provided you double-check it. To be sure, an excellent bedside manner can seldom make up for a lack of training, knowledge, and technical competence. But survivors have repeatedly told me there is a direct correlation between the confidence one has in one's health care team and one's probability of recovery. Communication skills shape that confidence level. You are seeking a balance here.

An Important Thing You Can Do

Evaluate your confidence level following an encounter with members of your medical team. This is particularly important when you are being asked to make treatment decisions. If you harbor more doubt than assurance toward your health care providers and their treatment recommendations, it is time to change either your confidence level or your team.

Be sure you are approaching this work at a comfortable pace. I suggest you take a break now and reflect on this important step. Continue your work after you have rested.

#9

Conviction Versus Wishful Thinking

Following an ovarian cancer diagnosis, Elaine, a busy mother and community volunteer, was told by her oncologist that an aggressive course of chemotherapy, one that would require hospitalization, was recommended.

Elaine deeply feared such a program. Still vivid in her memory was her mother-in-law's agonizing death from cancer. The side effects of her mother-in-law's chemotherapy treatment seemed worse than the illness. Elaine vowed at that time if she was ever diagnosed with cancer she would never have chemotherapy. Now she faced precisely the situation she feared most.

Elaine went in search of nontraditional treatments. Among others, she consulted a naturopath who suggested metabolic therapy, a combination of detoxification, herbs, and hyperthermia, the use of heat, to help destroy cancer cells. While this program sounded minimally toxic and noninvasive, Elaine now feared she was getting too far away from conventional medical care.

Then Elaine went to another medical oncologist. After she explained her fears and her search, this doctor recommended the use of hormones. Elaine was assured that hormonal therapy was typically less toxic than chemotherapy and in most cases generated far fewer side effects. But the hormone treatment was not as highly recommended as the original and more effective chemotherapy program.

Torn between these three different approaches, Elaine realized that the treatment she was most convinced would work was a combination of two. Through sheer persistence she was able to find an investigative technique that combined fractionated-dose chemotherapy with hyperthermia. On her own she adopted a nutritional supplementation program that included the herbs. She decided to hold the hormone treatment in reserve.

Elaine's choice of treatment is clearly not the answer for everyone. But following one's conviction is an important element of nearly every successful treatment program. Today, 11 years after her initial diagnosis, Elaine's cancer remains in remission, and she leads a full and happy life.

"I wanted conviction from my doctor," said Bill, a colon cancer survivor. "I looked him right in the eyes and asked, 'Is this treatment just the conventional thinking, Doctor? Or can you show me the hard data to back up your recommendation?' When he reviewed the PDQ recommendations, it seemed surgery followed by chemotherapy was my best bet."

An Important Thing You Can Do

Before you commit to a treatment program, take the time to ask some critical questions: "Do I really hold the belief that this is the right thing to be doing?" "Am I just taking the path of least resistance?" If you don't believe in it, resist! Find a treatment program that you can follow with conviction.

10

REFLECT
ON THE
TREATMENT
DECISION

If you've carefully read each step up to this point, you'll realize that you've simply been gathering information about treatment options. You have not yet made any treatment decisions. Now it is time to systematically review your treatment options one last time prior to crossing this Rubicon.

First, compare. Are you receiving consistent information from:

- The doctor who made the initial diagnosis?
- The oncologist whom you consulted for your second opinion?
- The recommendations you found through your independent research?

You should expect to see a reasonable consistency in the recommendations you receive from these sources. Most variances should relate to differences in levels of toxicity and degrees of invasiveness. If there is fundamental agreement, your decision-making process will probably be straightforward.

If the recommendations are inconsistent, then your information gathering is not complete. When you receive mixed signals, it is a certain sign to obtain a third qualified and independent opinion. This is time and money wisely spent.

Several prominent professionals in the oncology community have criticized me for this suggestion. Their objections have included: "The differences in treatment that you'll find are actually very minor." "You're just losing valuable time in receiving treatment." I disagree.

In all but the very rare case, the few days spent in gaining a third or fourth opinion are well worth the wait. As a patient you are after the very best treatment. You should expect a consistency of recommendations, if not a consensus.

Terry is a 47-year-old man from Indiana who was diagnosed with lymphoma. He obtained eight different opinions before agreeing to a program of treatment. Terry's determination to find the best has proven wise, and today he is alive and well.

Terry's experience points to an objection patients often raise: "But my insurance won't cover a third opinion." My response is, "Find a way." I was only too glad to pay for the services of qualified medical experts who would help determine the best course of treatment for me. Develop a similar attitude. Don't let insurance coverage limits determine this issue. Borrow the money or seek out a free clinic. There is nothing more important in your life at this moment.

Once you attain clarity and conviction in terms of the medical treatment, another evaluation needs a second reflective look. Are you comfortable with the people who will give you treatment and the place where the treatment will be administered?

June, a single mother in her fifties, had ovarian cancer. The treatment program in which she had the most confidence was recommended by doctors at a Comprehensive Cancer Center that was located more than an hour's commute away over busy California freeways. She was expected to visit the center weekly while undergoing treatment. The commute was a problem. June didn't want to drive in rush-hour traffic; a friend or family member would have to act as chauffeur. She also didn't feel completely safe in the part of the city where the center was located.

June expressed her concerns about the drive and her physical safety to the supervising oncologist. The doctor's response was compassionate and understanding. He was able to make arrangements at a hospital only ten minutes from June's apartment. She could receive her weekly treatments there and visit the cancer center just once a month. To this day, June believes the change in location was an important part of her successful recovery.

Does the recommended treatment program truly have your conviction? Are you convinced that the recommendations are the finest? Conviction implies a sense of certainty. While there are no guarantees, your treatment program and the people who administer it should elicit a strong degree of certainty that this is the right path to be taking at this time.

The Cancer Recovery Foundation of America has helped thousands of cancer patients walk through this treatment option analysis. Invariably the question arises, "What about all the alternative approaches? I really haven't checked them out." We have consistently recommended this strategy: First, explore the conventional treatment options. Surgery, radiation, and chemotherapy are the basis for the overwhelming majority of survivor success stories.

If the conventional treatment methods hold no real promise or are unsuccessful, then analyze both the investigative options, through National Cancer Institute–sponsored clinical trials, and the complementary and alternative therapies.

With all the options, integrate improved diet and nutritional supplementation, plus the psychosocial and psychospiritual techniques. Mobilize body, mind, and spirit. I believe that a physician who withholds this integrated treatment approach is no longer offering an informed medical opinion.

Allow yourself time to reflect on these important decisions. Don't be pressured by anyone to hurry a decision. When the treatment recommendations are consistent, the people who administer the treatment have your confidence, you understand the importance of integrating body, mind, and spirit, and you can say with conviction that this is what you should be doing now, then, and only then, are you ready to go to the next step.

An Important Thing You Can Do

Consult your notations in your Wellness and Recovery Journal. Thoughtfully, carefully, systematically, reflect on your treatment decision. Take another break. Reflect . . . again.

#11

DECIDE!

There is power in decision.

The cancer journey is made up of both little and big decisions. Your treatment program is a big one. In many ways it will determine the direction of your entire life. Now is the time to decide.

Decision is the spark that ignites action. Until a decision is reached, nothing happens.

Making decisions like this takes courage. But there is power in facing the fact that you have cancer, then carefully doing your homework, and finally choosing a course of action. Without exercising your courage, the problem will remain forever unaddressed.

Decide! Do not straddle the fence or make a partial decision. This is the time to take a firm stand on one side or another. Make a full commitment.

Yes, you will monitor your decision. You will keep your options open, of course. But now is the moment to say, "This is how we will climb the mountain! Now let's get started!"

Decision frees us from many of the uncertainties caused by

fear, doubt, and anxiety. Yes, there is risk. But there is greater risk in making no decision, hoping that all will magically be well.

Decide. You've done the work. This is not blind chance. This decision is the culmination of careful and sustained inquiry. Now is the time for action.

Decision awakens the spirit. Do you feel and sense that part of you springing to life? Nourish that spirit. Cherish it. It is the life force inside you working for you, helping you get well again.

Decide. The decision comes first, the results follow. Today is the day. Now is the hour. This is the moment! Decide!

An Important Thing You Can Do

Now, make the treatment decision. Appreciate the power of your commitment. Be optimistic. Decide! Inform your team of your choice.

#12

GIVE
ONLY
INFORMED
CONSENT

All treatment decisions should be made—must be made—with the informed consent of the patient or patient's guardian. This means you need to know in detail, in terms you can clearly understand, all the risks entailed in any procedure involving surgery, anesthesia, radiation therapy, chemotherapy, or similar medical encounter.

You'll be asked to sign a consent form. Do not sign a blank consent form. Make certain that the exact procedure is described and that you fully understand it. You have the right to set limits on these documents. You can cross out statements to which you do not consent. For example, I drew a line through the section of my consent form that asked my permission to videotape the operation for the removal of my lung.

You have the right to refuse treatment. An adult who is mentally competent can refuse treatment even if it may result in death. Nancy was a young woman who was pregnant. Even though she was advised to go ahead with treatment for lung cancer, she felt so strongly about the potential harm to her unborn child that she elected to postpone treatment until after her delivery. She exercised her right to refuse consent.

You need to understand clearly and completely all to which you are consenting. Gary, a retired pilot who made his home in Oregon, recognized that something was wrong with his health when he began to feel weak all the time. In six months he lost more than twenty pounds without dieting. "I just wasn't hungry," he said. "And I felt like I had a low-grade fever all the time." Then Gary became aware of swelling in his abdomen.

Finally he went to his doctor, who ordered a variety of tests. There was a complete physical examination, the most thorough he had ever experienced. Then came chest X rays, CAT scans, a blood workup, urine tests, and more. After consulting with other specialists, the doctor finally told Gary he had Hodgkin's disease.

Gary signed a consent form that said "laparotomy," thinking that he was giving permission for a biopsy. "The way it was presented," said Gary, "this seemed like just another test to determine, with more certainty, the extent of the disease. The doctor told me they needed to know where the cancer had spread. I thought it was no big deal and that I'd be out of the hospital the next day."

In fact, it was a big deal and Gary was not fully informed. A laparotomy is a surgical procedure that allows the doctors to explore the entire abdominal area. It is major surgery that should only be done by a team of experienced surgeons. Because of complications and infections, Gary's hospital stay lasted two and a half weeks. It left him with significant scars and lasting discomfort.

While Gary technically, even legally, gave consent to the procedure, in his mind he gave his okay for something much different. "I should have asked," lamented Gary. "But it seemed like no big deal."

Your doctor is obligated to inform you fully of any procedure to which you are being asked to give consent. This means explaining to you the procedure's purpose, risks, other alternatives, and the risk involved in not having the procedure. Don't be intimidated by the medical lingo. Make certain you get this information in language you understand. More important, make certain you ask detailed questions prior to giving any consent. Don't tolerate a physician's attitude that your concerns are unwelcome. If he or she is condescending or overly impatient, find another doctor. And be certain to include on your list of questions, "Why is this absolutely necessary?"

An Important Thing You Can Do

Ask your physician, not an associate, not an assistant, and not a nurse, to describe clearly the risks involved in your tests and treatment. Compare the risks to the expected benefits.

#13

BELIEVE IN YOUR TREATMENT PROGRAM

Excited belief is one of the great intangibles in a successful cancer treatment program. It is a natural extension of your conviction about your integrated treatment decisions. And it is your personal responsibility to believe in, and even be excited about, your treatment program.

Rachael and May both attended one of our Cancer Recovery Seminars in Atlanta. Rachael is a Georgia homemaker who started a course of radiation following surgery for breast cancer. Her attitude toward treatment was, "I guess it's something I have to do."

May received virtually the same diagnosis about a month after Rachael. May also had surgery and a follow-up course of chemotherapy. But her attitude was totally different from Rachael's: "I saw those chemicals as a great healing agent, something coming into my body to make me well. I welcomed my chemotherapy with open arms!"

Today May is free of cancer. Rachael continues to struggle.

Cancer survivors develop a confidence and an excited *belief* in their treatment programs that other patients do not possess. I am convinced that a correlation exists between belief in one's treatment and its effectiveness. My observations of the importance of belief in cancer treatment leads me to respect the awesome power of the mind and the human spirit in the cancer journey.

Colleen is a California wife, mother, and now retired elementary school teacher. After three years of remission, she had a recurrence of breast cancer including liver and bone metastasis. Her doctors gave her less than a year to live. "I knew I was at the crossroads," said Colleen. "And when I learned that survivors held an excited belief about their treatment, I decided I needed to do the same."

You can observe excited and expectant belief in survivor after survivor. I fully realize my observations are only anecdotal evidence and cannot stand up to scientific scrutiny. But I do not believe this hypothesis is wrong: Cancer survival is a matter of involving both head and heart. I have seen beliefs and attitudes like May's and Colleen's make the difference in hundreds of cases. To me the correlation between belief in treatment and effectiveness of treatment is very high.

Someday the scientific and medical communities will fully document the biological reality of this kind of optimism. In the meantime, I suggest you not enter the debate. Instead, learn from the survivors and develop an excited belief about your treatment.

An Important Thing You Can Do

"Own" your treatment program. See it as a friend. Believe it is there to help you. Excited belief is what you seek.

#14

OVERCOME NAUSEA

One of the realities for about half of the cancer patients under-going chemotherapy is nausea. While there are other side effects, the most common being hair loss, a feeling of tiredness, and the decreased ability of the body to make red and white blood cells and platelets, nausea is typically the most uncomfortable. It may or may not include vomiting.

Most people can significantly improve this experience, but it takes some experimentation. Here are some suggestions:

- Use relaxation exercises. (See #34)
- Eat smaller meals more often. Try six daily meals.
- Emphasize low-fat foods, especially fresh fruits.
- Limit liquids taken with meals. Drink no liquids in the hour before meals and the hour following meals. But be sure to take in enough liquids at other times. If you choose chemotherapy, your oncologist will tell you to drink more liquids to ensure good urine flow and minimize problems with liver, kidneys, and bladder.

- Clear cool liquids are recommended. Iced green tea, ginger ale, clear broths, popsicles, or apple juice ice cubes are worth trying. Take all liquids slowly.
- Eat dry food such as crackers, toast, popcorn—especially at the start of the day or at the first sign of nausea. Sorry, no butter on the popcorn.
- Eat salty foods. Avoid overly sweet foods.
- Do not lie down for two hours after eating. You can rest sitting up. Or if you simply must stretch out, prop a couple of pillows under your head to gain elevation.
- Sometimes loose clothing or fresh air will help in nausea control.
- Ask your pharmacist about Travel-Eze or Seaband anti-nausea wrist bands.
- Drink gingerroot tea steeped with peppermint.
- Goldenseal root may be helpful.
- Try hypnosis. Several small clinical trials have shown significant reductions in nausea and vomiting versus no hypnotherapy.
- Ask your oncologist for anti-nausea medication. Compazine, Tigan, and Zofran are commonly prescribed. Try taking them 30–60 minutes before treatment.

An Important Thing You Can Do

Clearly, there is no one-size-fits-all answer to nausea. You'll need to experiment with the suggested ideas. They have proven successful for many other cancer patients.

#15

MAKE THE MOST OF YOUR APPOINTMENTS

Free and open communication between you and your health care team is one of the most important aspects of your cancer recovery journey. You need to stay informed. You want feedback. But seldom is this information volunteered. You'll have to ask for it.

Wise patients bring a list of questions to virtually every medical appointment. If you have continuing or new symptoms, ask about them. If you are experiencing side effects, ask about them. Ask for further information about issues you have learned of from your reading or from talking to other patients.

"My radiation technician started to tease me about all my questions," said a retired Minneapolis professor who was being treated for prostate cancer. "I'd walk in the room and she'd say, 'What's on your list today, Dr. Nelson?' But I was determined to participate fully, to be an active patient. So I didn't let her remarks bother me in the least."

Speak with total honesty to your doctor and the entire health care team. They are not mind readers. Tell them your problems and ask for their opinions. Bring a family member with you if you have trouble being assertive. He or she can be your wellness advocate. Many people are intimidated by their doctors. If you are one of these people, recognize it and act immediately to remove that needless hurdle. If you are having trouble understanding and absorbing medical information, bring a tape recorder. Then you'll be able to review explanations and instructions at your convenience.

In case this hasn't been emphasized enough by now, please understand that your ability to ask questions is one of your most significant points of power. When in doubt, write down your questions and then read them from your list.

One other insider's tip: If you truly want to make the most of your medical appointments, get in the habit of expressing your sincere gratitude to your medical team. One of a group of doctors at a large health care system in Pittsburgh lamented to me, "We try so earnestly to help a patient. I wish once in a while they would simply say thank you." I clearly remember giving an appreciative hug to my oncologist. From that day forward I was treated like royalty in that office. Start showing your appreciation to these very important people in your life. Remember, they're people who respond to you just as you respond to them.

An Important Thing You Can Do

In your Wellness and Recovery Journal, record both your medical questions and the answers you are given. Keep this notebook handy. Bring it to your appointments. If you rely on your memory, or record your questions on bits of paper scattered here and there, you'll never have timely and accurate information.

Write a thank-you note to at least one person on your medical team following your next visit.

#16

MONITOR
YOUR
PROGRESS

As you continue your treatment program, you'll be given tests to determine how well it's working. Ask about the tests prior to agreeing to them. Then insist that the doctor share the results.

It's uplifting to know that you are making progress. But even a report that is less encouraging can have a positive side. It should lead you and your doctor to consider other forms of treatment. Many exist. If all standard therapies have been exhausted, perhaps now is the time to ask about investigative treatments, or to look more seriously at the complementary and alternative choices.

It is your responsibility to monitor your treatment program. Don't wait. Ask

An Important Thing You Can Do

Ask your doctor how and when he or she will check the progress of your treatment. Write this information in your Wellness and Recovery Journal. Then be certain tests occur as scheduled.

HEAL
YOUR
LIFESTYLE

A Stanford University health newsletter estimated that lifestyle issues such as poor diet, lack of exercise, and unwise general health habits accounted for 61 percent of the premature deaths due to cancer. They estimated the proportional contribution of genetics was 29 percent, and medical services themselves were listed as contributing to 10 percent of premature cancer deaths. The point is obvious: Lifestyle is critical in the survival journey.

Lifestyle issues are a matter of intentional choice. Clearly, there is much we can do to help ourselves get well again. Let's examine how thousands of cancer survivors have helped in their own healing.

#17

LIVE "WELL"

Wellness is an intentional choice of lifestyle, a way of living, a life stance that one chooses in order to maximize the enhancement of health and achieve the highest potential for total well-being.

Wellness is balance that encompasses body, mind, and spirit.

Wellness recognizes and acts on the fact that everything one thinks, says, does, feels, and believes has an impact on one's well-being.

Wellness can be chosen at any moment, in any circumstance. Wellness is possible with disability, regardless of physical condition.

For most people, "living well" typically means some major changes in lifestyle—in body, mind, and spirit.

We previously stated that cancer survivorship is a combination of head and heart. Conquering cancer demands that you reach beyond the physical issues of illness. Your mental, emotional, and spiritual health has a powerful effect on your well-being.

Kelly is a 48-year-old account executive with a major investment management firm. He developed malignant melanoma. "I went through the surgery and radiation just as recommended," said Kelly. "But I knew the real problem. I wasn't taking care of myself." Kelly hadn't exercised for years. His diet and nutrition habits were deplorable. He despised his work, and his marriage was coming apart.

Like so many survivors, Kelly considered cancer his wake-up call. "I realized my life was off course. And I knew it was up to me to change."

Similar sentiments are expressed by many survivors of cancer. They see illness as a message to make life changes. Kelly went on to reflect, "When I quit my job and opened a floral shop, my entire life started to heal. Cancer has actually been very good for me."

Living well, intentional choice, exercising the decision to take personal responsibility for one's total well-being—this is common talk among cancer survivors. It's whole-person wellness, a triumphant way of living without conditions.

Without conditions means that although wellness may be obscured by illness, it is a matter of personal choice whether wellness will be destroyed by illness. *Without conditions* means it is possible to discover high-level wellness in the very midst of life-threatening illness. Do not impose the condition of a "cure" on savoring the gift of life.

The decision to "live well" is significant and profound. Never again will your well-being be a static state measured simply by the lack of negative physical symptoms. Instead, wellness becomes your personal quest.

An Important Thing You Can Do

Begin the wellness quest. Open your mind and spirit to whole-person wellness. In your Wellness and Recovery Journal, record one step you can take today to improve your greater well-being. Now act, doing what is clearly doable today. Determine to live life at a new and higher level of wellness no matter what.

#18

OPERATE UNDER NEW ASSUMPTIONS

Compare the assumptions behind conventional health care with those behind whole-person wellness:

Assumptions behind conventional health care	Assumptions behind whole-person wellness
1. The patient is reliant upon the medical community.	1. The patient has, or should develop, independence.
2. The professional is the authority.	2. The professional is a healing partner.
3. Symptoms are treated, not investigated.	3. The underlying causes are sought, plus the symptoms are treated.
4. Specialized and concerned with body's subsystems.	4. Unified and concerned with person's whole life.
5. Body viewed as a series of mechanical functions.	5. Body viewed as a changing system.

Assumptions behind conventional health care	Assumptions behind whole-person wellness
6. Primary repairs made with surgery or drugs.	6. Intervention is minimal and appropriate. Noninvasive therapies are used when possible.
7. Pain and illness are purely negative.	7. Pain and illness are messages to value and act upon.
8. Mind and emotions are a secondary factor in health.	8. Mind and emotions are a major factor in health.
9. Body and mind are separate. Spirit has no health impact.	9. Body, mind, and spirit form one unit and always affect each other.
10. Disease prevention is largely environmental: not smoking, attention to diet, exercise, and rest.	10. Wellness means prevention plus wholeness: harmony in relationships, work, goals; a balance of body, mind, and spirit.

There is an important issue behind these assumptions. Your medical team will be helpful in addressing just one part of your cancer journey, the physical disease portion. Wellness encompasses far more. Whole-person well-being is our goal, the responsibility for achieving it falls to each of us personally.

An Important Thing You Can Do

Review the above assumptions. Circle those you believe to be true. Are you a traditionalist, or do you identify with the spirit of whole-person wellness? What does this analysis tell you to do differently? Which assumptions serve you best?

#19

Schedule Your Wellness

All important tasks demand a schedule. And there is no more important work in your life right now than the work of getting well again.

The trouble is, most people keep putting off the work of wellness, thinking they will get to it later. And guess what? They seldom, if ever, get around to it. Or if they do, it's only after everything else that is "important" has been accomplished.

Develop the attitude that there is nothing more important in your life right now than your work of wellness. For the time being, your wellness efforts need to take priority over family, job, community or religious activities, and social obligations. Getting well is your new top priority; you need to incorporate the disciplines of wellness into your daily life.

I actually blocked out my week on a schedule. Please turn the page and you'll see what a typical weekday looked like while I was in the middle of recovery:

6:00 A.M.	Wake up
6:15	Exercise
6:45	Meditate
7:00	Shower, eat, and commute
9:00	Work
Noon	Lunch and meditate
1:00 P.M.	Work
4:30	Commute
5:30	Meditate
6:00	Dinner
7:00	Family time
9:00	Read and meditate
10:00	Sleep

Doctors' appointments were worked in as needed. During commutes I virtually always listened to wellness tapes. Weekends found me devoting even more time to study and meditation. Throughout the entire process, I became more gentle with myself, demanding less in the way of outside activities and more in the way of self-care. I took control of my schedule and made the work of wellness my top priority.

An Important Thing You Can Do

Start a new page in your Wellness and Recovery Journal. Plan a schedule for your week similar to mine. Minimize obligations that cause undue stress. Give ample "core time" to the wellness disciplines discussed in this book.

> After completing your schedule, I suggest you take a break from your wellness work. Start the next section tomorrow or after you have rested. In the meantime, give careful consideration to how you spend your time. Do you understand I am asking you to make wellness a way of life? For most people, this means a major lifestyle shift. Look within. Consider the evidence and the implications of the suggestions. Begin now to modify your schedule to meet your new wellness priorities.

#20

ELIMINATE
ACTIVE
AND PASSIVE
SMOKING

It totally mystifies me how some cancer patients can continue to use tobacco. John had colon cancer. Following surgery, he started a course of chemotherapy. But do you think he quit smoking? No! "I don't have lung cancer," he'd say as he left our Cancer Recovery training sessions.

If I could communicate this any more strongly I would. If you are a user, cut out any and all tobacco immediately. Cigarettes, cigars, chewing tobacco—all must go. There is no excuse, even nicotine addiction, that is sufficient to continue this harmful habit that is putting cancer-causing chemicals into your body.

The question is not whether you can quit. The question is whether you will quit. I know this firsthand. I started smoking when I was in my teens. There is no doubt in my mind that smoking directly contributed to my lung cancer just over twenty years later. In those twenty years I seriously tried to quit five or six times. Willpower alone didn't get the job done. A change in thinking did.

It started with changing my self-perception. I first went from perceiving myself as a smoker to seeing myself as a person who chose the behavior of smoking. Seeing smoking as a behavior helped me detach emotionally and psychologically from the cigarettes. Then, I began to perceive myself as a nonsmoker. And in my mind, I told my smoking behavior to leave my life. This change in self-perception strategy can work for you, too.

In addition, eliminate your exposure to passive smoking. A Finnish study revealed up to a one-third drop in circulating levels of vitamin C and other antioxidants after just 30 minutes of exposure to secondhand smoke. Always sit in the nonsmoking sections. Ask your smoking co-worker to have his or her cigarette outside. You can take charge of this condition, too!

It has never been more important for you to maximize your health. Tobacco use and exposure to secondhand smoke have no place in the quest for wellness.

An Important Thing You Can Do

Stop all tobacco use immediately. Wean yourself with a nicotine patch if you need to. Stay away from tobacco users while they are smoking.

#21

ADOPT THIS DIETARY STRATEGY DURING TREATMENT

There has never been a more important time in your life to eat well. Cancer can deplete the body's nutrients and cause weight loss. Cancer and cancer treatments can also have a negative effect on appetite as well as the body's ability to digest foods. The result is a dilemma—high nutrient need and low nutrient intake.

Scientific evidence of diet's link with cancer recovery is overwhelming. But nutritional therapy is not well understood by most traditional health care providers. "Why doesn't my doctor tell me about this?" is a common question of cancer patients. It reflects an erroneous cultural mindset—all health information must flow from the "authority," which usually means the doctor.

In fact, if you look to your oncologist for information and positive reinforcement regarding nutrition as a cancer therapy, you will most likely be disappointed. The reason is generally a lack of knowledge rather than an antinutrition bias; medical education simply puts little emphasis on nutrition.

In order to optimize your cancer recovery potential, your body demands premium-grade fuel. Your dietary and nutritional habits can make a significant contribution to your getting well again. While individualized nutritional plans are recommended, here's a winning strategy that has proven successful for thousands of cancer survivors.

1. Maintain a Healthy Weight

Quality of weight (muscle versus fat) is a more important indicator than the number of pounds on the scale. Maintain a diet that is high enough in calories to keep up your normal healthy body weight. Prior to beginning treatment, make it your goal to gain 5 or 10 pounds. You'll do well to build these reserves. This is no time to start a crash diet. Weigh yourself each week and record the results in your journal.

2. Emphasize Protein

Eat foods that are high in protein. The best sources are nonfat dairy foods, grains, legumes, seeds, and nuts. You can also obtain low-fat protein from beans and fish. I also consume eight ounces of nonfat yogurt daily. It not only contains protein but also lactobacillus acidophilus, which helps improve the presence of beneficial bacteria in the intestines. Your protein and calorie needs are greater during treatment and recovery than normal. Emphasizing low-fat, mostly vegetable protein will help keep your energy level high, maintain strength, and rebuild normal tissue affected by treatments.

3. Increase Food Quality

Eat "live" premium foods, those that are minimally processed, in as close to their natural state as possible. Valuable nutrients, including fiber, vitamins, and minerals, are often removed from refined foods. Refined foods often contain excessive amounts of fat, salt, and preservatives. Your first choice: fresh fruits, fresh vegetables, and whole grains. If a food is boxed, bottled, canned, or frozen, it has most often been processed and lacks the "live" nutritional content of the fresh alternative.

An Important Thing You Can Do

Determine that during treatment you will eat better than you have in your entire life. The strategy: maintain weight, eat plenty of protein, and choose "live" premium foods.

#22

FOLLOW
THESE
"EAT SMART"
GUIDELINES

Unless your physician has prescribed a special diet, there are "eat smart" guidelines that you would be wise to follow in overcoming your cancer:

- When in doubt, eat a plant. Fresh fruits and fresh vegetables are now your foods of choice.
- Eat breads and pastas that are made from whole grains.
- Look to beans and legumes for protein. Try brown rice with any type of bean. Obtain additional protein by sprinkling chopped nuts or soy nuts over steamed vegetables and fresh salads.
- Eliminate red meats. Limit chicken and turkey. "Flesh foods" are difficult to digest fully and have been linked by some researchers to stomach, bladder, liver, breast, and colon cancers.
- If you must have animal protein, try water-packed tuna and steamed or broiled fish.
- Use low-fat or nonfat dairy products. Even some cheeses and ice creams are now made with low-fat or nonfat milk.

- Use monosaturated fats like canola and olive oils whenever possible. If you must fry foods, use a nonstick spray.
- Use fat- and sugar-reduced products whenever possible. Limit consumption of foods with fat and sugar substitutes.
- Eat very few risky foods. Consume caffeine and alcoholic beverages, and salt-cured, pickled, and smoked foods in strict moderation.

There are specific foods and nutrients that help you heal. Start now to plan your meals, both those eaten at home as well as those where you dine out, around the natural nutrient-rich foods in each of the following categories:

Vitamin A/Carotenoids

A variety of studies suggest that vitamin A and its relatives, especially beta and mixed carotene, contain anti-cancer properties. Several studies show evidence that diets high in carotenoids or vitamin A lower the risk of cancer of the esophagus, larynx, and lung. A Finnish study did show increased risk of lung cancer among male smokers who consumed beta-carotene. The findings were confirmed by a larger trial. So, if you smoke, the evidence says no beta-carotene. For nonsmokers, the studies also indicate a protective effect in precancerous changes in the prostate, bladder, and breast. Some dosage intelligence is required: Vitamin A is liver toxic in high doses; carotenoids found in fruits and vegetables are not. Foods high in vitamin A/carotenoid content include:

Apricots	Broccoli	Spinach	Papaya
Butternut squash	Red peppers	Sweet potatoes	Peaches
Chard	Collard greens	Skim milk	Pumpkin
Cantaloupe	Carrots	Oranges	Mangos

VITAMIN C

Fewer cancers of the stomach and esophagus occur in people whose diets emphasize citrus fruits and vegetables that are rich in vitamin C. What is not clear, however, is whether vitamin C or some of the bioflavinoid components of the C-containing foods are the protective factor. Initial studies indicate that vitamin C may also combat genetically induced colon polyps, which often lead to colon cancer. Foods high in vitamin C include:

Broccoli	Cabbage	Collard greens	Kiwi
Papaya	Red peppers	Sweet potatoes	Brussels sprouts
Cantaloupe	Grapefruit	Mangos	Peas
Rutabagas	Turnip greens	Tangerines	Cauliflower
Kale	Oranges	Potatoes	Lemons and limes

CALCIUM

Studies indicate a link between higher calcium intake and lower rates of intestinal cancer. Higher calcium consumption is also associated with reduced risk of osteoporosis. Foods high in calcium include:

Broccoli	Collard greens	Salmon	Nonfat cheese
Tofu	Great northern	Figs (dried)	Nonfat yogurt
Kale	beans	Sardines	

CRUCIFEROUS VEGETABLES

Studies show that eating vegetables from the cabbage family may reduce the incidence of gastrointestinal cancers. Cruciferous vegetables include:

Broccoli	Cauliflower	Turnips	Brussels sprouts
Kale	Cabbage	Rutabagas	

Vitamin E

Several studies indicate that high intake of vitamin E may stimulate immune function. Other studies show that low blood levels of vitamin E are linked to increased risk of lung, colon, and rectal cancers. Foods high in vitamin E:

Cabbage	Collard greens	Olive oil	Canola oil
Kale	Wheat germ	Chard	Mangos

Fiber

Diets high in fiber are linked with lower rates of colon cancer. The recommended daily fiber intake is 30 to 40 grams. Foods high in fiber include:

Apricots	Brown rice	Cabbage	Cauliflower
Figs	Kale	Mangos	Peas
Prunes	Rutabagas	Turnips	Bran cereal
Chard	Oranges	Broccoli	Butternut
Kidney beans	Wheat germ	Beans (black	squash
Strawberries	Collard greens	and pinto)	Kiwi
Carrots	Potatoes	Sweet potatoes	Whole grain
Papaya	Cantaloupe	Grapefruit	bread
Brussels sprouts	Popcorn	Pumpkin	

Selenium

Some studies indicate that high levels of selenium may lower cancer risk. Selenium may have a protective effect against breast and colon cancer. Foods high in selenium:

Brown rice	Tuna	Oatmeal
Swordfish	Whole grain breads	Skinless chicken
Salmon	Whole grain cereal	breast

Low Fat

Studies clearly show that excessive fat intake increases the risk of developing cancer of the breast, colon, and prostate. A high-fat diet contributes to obesity, which has also been linked to cancer of the uterus, gallbladder, breast, and colon. Nearly 40 percent of calories consumed by Americans come from fat. The level should be limited to no more than 20 percent of caloric intake. Foods low in fat:

Nonfat milk	All cereals and grains
Nonfat cheese	All vegetables except avocados
Nonfat yogurt	All bread except biscuits and
All fruits	croissants

An Important Thing You Can Do

For one week, keep a food diary in your Wellness and Recovery Journal. Record all foods and beverages you consume. Be precise. Compare your diet with the above guidelines. Where is there room for improvement? Emphasize the "eat smart" guidelines in your diet.

#23

REPLACE
FLUIDS

Are you looking for a simple action that will vastly increase your opportunity for survival and recovery? Here it is: Drink the equivalent of eight cups of water each and every day! Not coffee. Not soda. Not juice. Water.

It is an almost universal truth—people with cancer are dehydrated. Lack of water inhibits immune function, the most potent defense you have against cancer. The environment your cells live in is not blood, it is fluid. The lymph system, a key component of your immune system, is a fluid system requiring adequate water to function at its highest capacity.

Through natural elimination, perspiration, and even breathing, your body loses water daily. Fluid must be continually replaced in appropriate quantities for you to be optimally well.

I prefer water with no chlorine or fluorides. This is difficult to obtain from most municipal water systems. Even bottled water, especially if contained in plastic, is not a sure answer. Some research indicates that sunlight starts a chemical reaction in the plastic bottle that can result in carcinogens in the water.

How can you get pure water? I recommend a water purification system in your home or certified, chemical-free, spring-fed bottled water in glass containers.

An Important Thing You Can Do

Drink eight cups of pure water each day.

#24

KNOW WHY YOU'RE EATING

Long-term dietary changes require more than shifts in our menus. Our food preferences are a factor of culture and habit. Our enjoyment of food is so much a part of our lives that any permanent change must involve not only *what* we eat but also *why* we eat.

On countless occasions we allow our frame of mind, rather than our bodies, to determine our food choices. Comfort foods to satisfy our emotions, to soothe our anger, frustration, worry, boredom, or guilt, are most often the culprit. Relief from emotional distress is easily accomplished by eating. When this happens we have linked diet to emotional fulfillment. This is dangerous territory.

We need a heightened awareness of why we eat. Many patients who embark on the cancer recovery journey develop an attitude that changing their diet is something they have to do, which is too bad. I suggest you try an outlook that reflects the fact that a change in diet is something you get to do!

Eating with awareness is easily accomplished with the help of these proven practices:

- Don't keep any high-fat snack foods around the house where they will be a serious temptation.
- Make a rule of not eating in front of the television, where you don't pay attention to what or how much you eat.
- Don't eat so quickly that you can't enjoy your food. It takes about twenty minutes for our brains to realize that our stomachs are full. Slow down. Take a break mid-meal.
- Reward appropriate eating behavior, but don't use comfort foods as the reward. If you've had a good week or have reached a wellness goal, treat yourself to a movie, a concert, or a new outfit. Don't punish imperfection, just don't reward yourself. Try again next week.
- Make each meal a pleasant experience. Stop eating on the run or while standing at the kitchen counter. Take time to put out a place setting. Offer a short affirmation or prayer of gratitude for each meal. You'll then be nurturing yourself emotionally and spiritually, as well as physically.

An Important Thing You Can Do

Distinguish between a food craving, which is a psychological need, and hunger, which is the body's need for nourishment. Check your urge to eat the next time you see a food advertisement. A craving diminishes when we take on another activity. Go for a walk. Call a friend. Read a book. Then evaluate. Were you feeling a craving or hunger? Honor your hunger, not your craving. Eat with awareness!

#25

Determine Your Vitamin, Mineral, and Herbal Supplements

Most cancer survivors believe in and use vitamin and mineral supplements. Many also employ herbs as nutritional therapy. It is encouraging to see many more health care professionals endorse nutritional supplementation.

The goal of supplementation is to support maximum immune function, to build up the host organism so that it is able to cope with the challenge that it is facing. Nutritional supplements are an outstanding choice in this effort. But, to keep supplementation in proper perspective, it is essential to emphasize that survivors typically consume vitamins, minerals, and herbs in addition to, not in place of, implementing conventional treatment approaches. Also, these supplements are used in addition to, not in place of, the anti-cancer "eat smart" guidelines previously discussed.

Once I understood how widespread supplementation was, I decided to follow suit. But each patient is responsible for his or her own decisions on this issue. The problem is, the whole field of nutritional supplementation has an uncertain reputation. Just like some of the conventional treatment choices, there is a dearth of solid research. As you explore this subject, you'll find some people making incredible unsubstantiated claims that just do not stand up to scientific scrutiny. So be very careful, even skeptical.

I was helped by a nutritional therapist. After much study and consultation, I adopted the following supplementation program:

Supplement	Daily Dose
Beta-carotene	25,000 IU
Vitamin C (powdered)	10,000 mg
Vitamin E	400 IU
Vitamin B complex	50 mg
Folic acid	400 μg
Pantothenic acid	50 mg
Potassium	500 mg
Selenium	50 μg
Zinc	30 mg

During the time of my radiation treatments, I also added garlic capsules at the equivalent dosage of 3,000 μg of allicin per day.

I stress that this was *my* approach. These are not specific recommendations for any individual. In fact, I may have been ill-advised. Certainly some changes would be called for given today's better understanding of supplementation. Those changes follow. Most important, I want to guide your attention to a group of vitamins and minerals known as the "antioxidants" as well as six different herbs that are in wide use with cancer treatments, particularly outside the United States. Then you can make your own decisions.

ANTIOXIDANT VITAMINS AND MINERALS

Antioxidants are believed to protect the body's cells and tissues from oxidative damage which may cause normal cells to become cancerous. Antioxidants may also stimulate the immune system and improve resistance to tumor growth. These supplements should be consumed with food, not alone, as this will help improve absorption.

Vitamin A and Mixed Carotenoids

The first component of antioxidant supplements is the vitamin A family, including the carotenoids. Mixed carotenoids are safer than vitamin A supplements, which may be toxic at high doses. The body converts carotenoids into vitamin A only when it is needed.

Therapeutic supplementation:
Recommended daily dosage of beta and mixed carotenes is 25,000 IU per day.

Cautions:
Slightly orange skin discoloration in the palms of your hands is a sign you have reached the point of maximum dosage.

Vitamin C (Ascorbic Acid)

Vitamin C is an antioxidant that protects lipids (fats) and cell membranes from oxidation. It may also protect the lungs from damage caused by smoke and ozone. Vitamin C may also work synergistically with vitamin E, another antioxidant. Studies also indicate that vitamin C may enhance both chemotherapy and radiation effects. Japanese research indicates vitamin C can block damage to heart muscles that often occurs when doctors treat patients with highly toxic cancer treatment drugs like Adriamycin and interleukin-2.

Therapeutic supplementation:
Recommended daily dosage range is 2 to 12 grams per day.

Cautions:
You will need to build to this level as too much vitamin C taken too quickly will lead to diarrhea. Should this occur, reduce

dosage by half for 48 hours and then resume the build-up. Your body will eventually and naturally tell you its vitamin C requirements. I recommend powdered vitamin C.

Vitamin E (Tocopherol)

Vitamin E is the primary fat-soluble antioxidant. It works in tandem with selenium to block oxidation of polyunsaturated fats that make up cell membranes. Vitamin E may stimulate the immune system as well as enhance radiation therapy and protect healthy cells from the effects of chemotherapy.

Therapeutic supplementation:
Recommended daily dosage is now 800 to 1,200 IU during recovery.

Cautions:
Vitamin E may be linked to high blood pressure in a small percentage of individuals. If you have high blood pressure, a history of heart disease, or diabetes, begin vitamin E supplements at 50 IU per day. Increase the daily dose by 50 IU every week until you reach the desired dose level.

Selenium

This is a naturally occurring trace mineral and part of an important enzyme called glutathione peroxidase, which protects tissue from oxidative damage of free radicals generated by smoke, smog, ultraviolet light, radiation, alcohol, and other environmental toxins. Selenium is found naturally in seafood, meat, and, in smaller amounts, in whole grains.

Therapeutic supplementation:
Recommended dosage is 200–400 µg per day.

Cautions:
Selenium is toxic at levels above 2,000 µg per day.

Herbal Supplementation

Herbs are used with increasing frequency by cancer survivors. Of course, herbs and spices have been used medicinally for thousands of years. Many conventional medicines were originally derived from herbs. Six herbs are used extensively in the treatment of cancer outside the United States. I ask that you consider these in your own recovery program.

Milk Thistle (Cardus Marianus)

A liver-protective antioxidant and immune stimulant. Especially important for those who choose chemotherapy. Also used for hepatitis and cirrhosis.

Therapeutic supplementation: 200 mg twice daily.

Cautions: None

Echinacea (Echinacea Angustifolia)

Used for viral infections, wound healing, and as an immune stimulant. German government commission recommends four weeks on, one week off.

Therapeutic supplementation: 1,200 mg three times daily.

Cautions: None

Astragalus (Astragalus Membranaceous)

Immune stimulant.

Therapeutic supplementation: 400 mg three times daily.

Cautions: None

Garlic (Allium Sativum)

Used for cardiac disease as it lowers LDL cholesterol. Garlic also inhibits platelet aggregation, which lowers metastatic opportunities.

Therapeutic supplementation: 1 or 2 fresh cloves daily, or equivalent of 4,000 µg allicin daily.

Cautions: Do not use while taking prescription anticoagulants. Diarrhea is possible at high dosage.

Ginger (Zingiber Officinale)

Anti-inflammatory, anti-emetic, and anti-spasmodic. Especially helpful for control of nausea.

Therapeutic supplementation: 1 to 2 grams three times daily, or ginger tea as needed.

Cautions: High dosage may lead to miscarriage. Double dosage for inflammations.

Ginseng Siberian (Eleutherococcus Senticosus)

Lowers cholesterol and blood pressure. Enhances immune function.

Therapeutic supplementation: 1 to 3 capsules daily, or tea, 1 to 3 cups daily.

Cautions: Large doses can cause insomnia, diarrhea, and skin lesions.

OTHER OPTIONAL SUPPLEMENTS

I became convinced that even more supplementation was appropriate for me. The cancer-fighting evidence on dietary fiber is significant. In essence, a clean colon leads to improved health—the same view that metabolic alternative therapies adopt. I began the daily intake of 45 to 50 grams of fiber, consuming equal amounts of wheat, oat, and psyllium brans. Twice daily I consume half the bran, along with powdered vitamin C and a tablespoon of liquid calcium magnesium citrate, mixed in orange juice. The net effect is to create a cleansing and detoxification program. It's oral chelation. This seems right for me.

I urge you to constantly monitor research on vitamin, mineral, and herbal supplementation. An especially promising catalytic antioxidant is Coenzyme Q10 (CoQ10). In a Danish study, CoQ10 was linked to regression of breast cancer. Even though the scientific investigation is at an early stage, you may wish to consider CoQ10 as a supplement if you are diagnosed with breast cancer. The Danish study prescribed a daily oral dose of 390 mg. Supporting literature indicates doses up to 300 mg daily should produce no side effects.

I also encourage you to follow the research on the hormone melatonin. Early studies indicate melatonin in conjunction with radiation therapy may prolong survival time and improve quality of life in people with brain cancers. Early evidence of melatonin's effectiveness has also been seen in colon, rectal, and breast cancers. Melatonin has also been linked with increased immune activity following surgery. If you choose to supplement with melatonin, I encourage you to do so in very small doses. Forthcoming research will more accurately set dosage guidelines.

In addition to the Quillins' book recommended in #29, I recommend the serious student of nutrition study *Prescription for Nutritional Healing* by James F. Balch, M.D. and Phyllis A. Balch, C.N.C. for complete information on the therapeutic use of vitamins, minerals, herbs, and food supplements.

An Important Thing You Can Do

Telephone a professional nutritionist. Ask what experience he or she has in therapeutic nutritional supplementation for cancer recovery. If indicated, make an appointment for a consultation. Compare those recommendations with your own research. Make your supplement decisions based on the same standards you used for conventional treatments.

#26

MAKE EXERCISE PART OF YOUR RECOVERY PROGRAM

Hundreds of cancer survivors helped me make an important discovery: Exercise directly correlates with health recovery. Nine out of ten people I interviewed talked about keeping physically active. Even people who were incapacitated or who needed a wheelchair emphasized their commitment to a regular exercise program.

Cancer survivors are markedly different, however, in their exercise goals. Very few set out to run a marathon or become Olympic athletes. Instead, the most common exercise goal among cancer survivors is to experience an increase in energy.

I chose walking as my exercise. At first I was so weak that even a couple of minutes of walking was too much. So I began with chair exercises doing simple arm circles—the backstroke movement with my arms fully extended. I'd do ten sets clockwise and follow with ten sets in the reverse direction. Soon I felt that increase in energy—the deeper breathing, the increase in heart rate, and the better skin color.

It wasn't long before I began to feel stronger. It seemed exercise was working! So I added a few minutes of leg lifts. Soon I was strong enough to put walking back into my exercise routine. Initially, I walked for perhaps five minutes before feeling an increase in energy. But soon that time stretched to 10 minutes. Over the months the exercise periods became longer. I bought an exercise book and added some full-body stretching routines before the start of my walk, and I ended the exercise session with some light calisthenics. I began to feel the combination of physical and emotional regeneration working together to enhance my well-being. You can experience the same.

Today I believe I have found the right balance. Hardly a day passes that I do not walk for at least 30 minutes. I precede the walk with about three minutes of full-body stretches and conclude the session with five minutes of push-ups and sit-ups.

This did not happen overnight. I determined this to be my correct level over a period of two years. Several times I have experimented with exercise beyond the normal 35-to-40-minute daily routine. I tried walking for an hour each day but found I was experiencing hip soreness. I tried weight lifting only to realize I didn't enjoy it.

Some people think more exercise is better. A gentleman recently wrote me to express his opinion that two hours of intense exercise each day is a requirement for cancer recovery. I don't recommend it. Between the threat of injury associated with extended exercise and the rigid, grinding routine that often results in burnout, I believe more harm than good can come from workouts that last two or three hours daily.

Instead, I recommend you find a type of exercise that you enjoy. Then practice that routine just until you feel an increase in energy. The physical benefits will include increased flexibility, greater strength, more cardiovascular capacity, weight loss, and lower blood pressure. But the psychological benefits are even greater—joy, enthusiasm, and mental vitality. What a payoff!

Make exercise part of your cancer recovery program. No matter how long it has been since you have exercised, no matter how incapacitated or confined you are, there are exercises you can do. Exercise will help you get well again.

An Important Thing You Can Do

After an okay from your doctor, exercise just until you feel an increase in energy. This is your only exercise goal. Do the same tomorrow. Keep extending the duration as you build strength and stamina. No more excuses! Take charge. Your body will respond to your "get-well" signals.

#27

GET
MORE
SLEEP

"I'm always so tired. My radiation treatments drain me," noted Olivia during her recovery from breast cancer. "I just want to sleep all the time. But with all my responsibilities, who has time to sleep?"

Fatigue is part of nearly every cancer patient's experience. Unfortunately, many patients interpret fatigue as an indication of their fast-approaching demise. This is not necessarily so.

During and just after treatment, you are a different person physically. Just consider what is happening to you. With surgery, a major wound has been inflicted on your body. Chemotherapy puts chemicals into your system that alter your unique biochemical makeup. Radiation causes genetic and cellular changes in your body. Repairs demand rest. No wonder cancer patients are tired.

"For three months I cut back to half days at work," said Ted after his bout with bladder cancer. "I took an afternoon nap for a year following my treatment," shared Alicia, who recovered from ovarian cancer. "I still take afternoon naps," said Bert, celebrating his six-year anniversary of a lung cancer diagnosis.

The fact is, survivors rest. It is a major mistake to carry on at the same frantic pace to which you were accustomed when you were supposedly healthy. Feeling tired is normal for anyone with any illness. During treatment you may feel tired for weeks until your body gets the opportunity to adjust and recover. So allow yourself rest.

Provided you are getting adequate food and moderate exercise, fatigue is nothing to consume you with worry. It is not a sure sign of your demise. Take that morning nap. Add an afternoon nap if you require it. Or a short rest before dinner may be just what is needed. Eight or more hours of sleep each night is an absolute essential.

An Important Thing You Can Do

Give yourself permission to get more sleep. Block out rest times on your wellness schedule. Allow your body the rest it needs to repair and heal.

#28

FIND A
POSITIVE
SUPPORT
GROUP

You need a support group. Consider this evidence: Cancer patients who regularly attend support group meetings live longer than those who do not.

Ongoing research at Stanford University confirmed what cancer survivors have known for decades. In a study of patients with advanced breast cancer, those who attended a weekly two-hour support group session had a life expectancy twice that of the nonattenders. Further research at U.C.L.A. and King's College in London confirms the value of attending support groups. The message is clear: We truly need one another for survival.

Distinguish between the two major types of support groups: informational and psychosocial. The informational groups communicate basic knowledge on a wide variety of oncology issues. Subjects might include types of cancer treatments, common side effects, physical therapy following breast surgery, or how to live with an ostomy. The idea behind this type of support group is simply to inform.

More critical to survival are the psychosocial support groups.

These are the supportive/expressive therapeutic programs that focus on the emotional, psychological, and spiritual aspects of cancer. Look for groups that take a stance of hope without denying the reality of the illness. At meetings you should expect to express your own fears and frustrations freely and allow others in the group to do the same. You'll learn from the responses of the group members who have overcome cancer, and you'll contribute to those who are just beginning the cancer recovery journey.

One warning: A potential problem with any type of support group is that instead of encouraging personal growth, many groups quickly turn into a "pity party." While there is significant value in allowing people to talk out their problems, the discerning group needs a leader to judge when the talking is therapeutic and when it is rehearsing, and reinforcing, a problem. The "cyber-solace" provided in on-line chat groups is no exception.

When a group of us started Cancer Conquerors support groups, committing to support one another in our wellness quests, we made a pact early on. Each meeting would include a lesson— somebody leading a discussion on a recovery principle—and a time for open discussion and support. The emphasis was to be on the application of lessons that would help contribute to our own healing. It was the smartest move we ever made. We have experienced very few pity parties.

An Important Thing You Can Do

Contact Cancer Recovery Foundation of America or check with your oncologist. Attend several types of support groups. Judge for yourself. Are they actively working toward wellness or conducting a pity party?

If you don't find what you are looking for, perhaps you need to consider starting a group in your home. Thousands of patients have done so, benefiting themselves and others in their community. Contact Cancer Recovery Foundation of America for start-up information. You'll find the contact information on page 170.

HEAL
WITH THE
MIND

Do personal beliefs, positive attitudes, and hopeful expectations make a contribution to cancer recovery? Credible scientific evidence says, "Yes." In fact, the contribution may be greater than we ever imagined.

Fighting cancer is much more than simply excising a tumor, treating a malignancy with radiation, or injecting chemotherapy into a vein. Think of harnessing all your resources, including the mind, in the quest for survival. The basics are really quite simple. Let's continue our work.

#29

READ AND
STUDY
THESE
BOOKS

Knowledge is power. Educate yourself! Obtain these books and start to study:

American Cancer Society. *Informed Decisions: The Complete Book of Cancer Diagnosis, Treatment, and Recovery.* New York: Viking, 1997. If you don't have access to the world wide web, this is the book for information on conventional medical approaches.

Anderson, Greg. *The Cancer Conqueror.* Dallas: Word, 1988/Andrews & McMeel, 1990. My thoughts, experience, and encouragement to readers on how to integrate body, mind, and spirit.

Benson, Herbert and Miriam Klipper. *The Relaxation Response.* New York: Avon, 1976. The definitive source for relaxation and meditation concepts and techniques.

Borysenko, Joan. *Minding the Body, Mending the Mind.* Reading, MA: Addison-Wesley, 1987. How to manage stress and uncertainty and find workable solutions.

Korda, Michael. *Man to Man: Surviving Prostate Cancer.* New York: Vintage, 1997. Excellent update on the latest treatment options. Straight talk from a man who has been there.

Lerner, Michael. *Choices in Healing: Integrating the Best of Conventional and Complementary Approaches to Cancer.* Cambridge, MA: MIT Press, 1996. This book is the intellectual's guide to alternative treatments.

LeShan, Lawrence. *Cancer as a Turning Point.* New York: Plume, 1994. The emotional aspects of cancer. Contains exercises involving reflection, discussion, and writing to help come to terms with fears.

Love, Susan M. *Dr. Susan Love's Breast Book.* Reading, MA: Addison-Wesley, 1995. Excellent discussion of breast health including treatment options and expected outcomes.

Morra, Marion, and Eve Potts. *Choices: Alternatives in Cancer Treatment.* New York: Avon, 1994. Comprehensive questions and answers about cancer treatment. Excellent resource listings.

Quillin, Patrick and Noreen. *Beating Cancer with Nutrition* (Revised). Tulsa: Nutrition Times, 1998. Excellent scientifically backed research and recommendations on nutrition as complementary therapy.

Siegel, Bernie. *Love, Medicine, and Miracles.* New York: Harper & Row, 1986. Stories about self-healing from a former surgeon's observations of cancer patients and support group work.

Simonton, O. Carl, Stephanie Matthews-Simonton, and James Creighton. *Getting Well Again.* New York: Bantam, 1978. Guides cancer patients to participate in recovery through imagery and psychotherapy.

An Important Thing You Can Do

Visit your bookstore or library. Conduct your own research. Become an expert on your illness and especially on your pathway to wellness.

#30

DISCOVER YOUR BELIEFS

Literally thousands of cancer survivors radically change their beliefs about cancer and about life. Many consider this to be the most fundamental aspect of healing with the mind. I believe this idea has a central place in your own recovery efforts.

Attitudes have to do with one's state of mind, with one's mental habits. Beliefs are something different; now we are talking about convictions, the implications of certainty surrounding mental positions.

There are three widely held beliefs that work against overcoming cancer:

1. A diagnosis of cancer means my certain death.
2. The treatment program for cancer is drastic, is of questionable effectiveness, and involves many unpleasantries.
3. This situation "just happened" to me and therefore there is little I can do to influence it.

All of these beliefs are untrue! The truth about these statements is:

1. Cancer, no matter how advanced, may or may not mean death.
2. A wide range of treatments do exist. They have the potential to be effective. The difficulties in recovery are far outweighed by the benefits.
3. Most illnesses do not "just happen." On several levels, our ability to influence health, either positively or negatively, is at work.

These truths can work for you in your recovery. Your response to a problem is more powerful than the problem itself. There is much you can do.

Do beliefs actually affect recovery? Consider this. Beliefs and expectations constantly contribute to actual experience in all areas of life, including the experience of cancer. If we believe a rainy day means gloom, gloom is what we experience.

I realize it's a long way from rainy days to cancer recovery. But this much is clear: Beliefs can be changed and chosen. The trouble is, we seldom consciously choose them. Perhaps beliefs have simply been accepted by us for many years, like the conventional wisdom surrounding cancer. Perhaps we had beliefs imposed from parents, co-workers, or friends. We may have picked up other people's beliefs and made them our own. They may or may not be true or helpful. But these beliefs have significant power.

Awareness of our fundamental beliefs is often the first, and certainly one of the most dramatic ways to improve our circumstances. If you are harboring the belief that cancer means death, challenge it! The fact is, there are long-term survivors of every type of cancer, including many patients who have been told by doctors that there was no hope.

An Important Thing You Can Do

Analyze your beliefs. In your Wellness and Recovery Journal, complete the following sentences with the first thoughts/feelings that come to mind:

1. When I think of my cancer diagnosis, my thought is_____

_____

2. I believe my cancer treatment is_____

_____

3. The one thing I believe would best help me is_____

_____

Analyze how your beliefs align with the truth. Talk to others who have successfully traveled the cancer journey. Discover what they believe. Vow to change your self-limiting beliefs today.

#31

"Reframe"
Your
Cancer

If you're like most cancer patients, you look upon your illness as the most overwhelming threat to life you've ever encountered. "I thought of cancer as a powerful evil force inflicting great injury on me," said Raymond, a retired restaurant owner who was battling cancer of the larynx. "It was the ultimate threat."

Raymond's words describe his mental outlook. *Cancer . . . a powerful evil force . . . inflicting great injury . . . the ultimate threat.* It took weeks of counseling, but Raymond came to view his cancer not as a threat but as a challenge. Cancer became something that stimulated him to introspection, to review his life. Raymond ultimately made changes in his exercise routine, diet, job, and spiritual life. Cancer became Raymond's wake-up call.

Raymond's experience is a perfect example of what it means to reframe the illness. Reframing is the process of finding alternative ways, more positive means, of viewing and responding to any circumstance.

Jose's diagnosis of prostate cancer was the most frightening and unwelcome event in his 58 years. Even though tests confirmed that the cancer had been discovered early and the prognosis was quite optimistic, his chronic panic-driven thought process focused on his imminent demise. "I didn't just have cancer, I was cancer," said Jose.

Frank also had prostate cancer, but his was significantly more advanced than Jose's. Frank had bone involvement. Unlike Jose, Frank made the critical distinction that he had cancer, the cancer did not have him. "I realized that my mind and spirit had cancer only if I allowed it." Frank's outlook reframed the cancer.

Frank's response demonstrates the significant power we possess. The point of control is not the circumstance of illness so much as our response to the illness. Our response can make all the difference. When we reframe cancer, we respond differently and more proactively. We acknowledge and nourish our inner strength, even in the face of doubt and fear. The threat subsides. We take on the challenge.

Fortunately, both stories have happy endings. Jose was able to embrace many of Frank's more positive beliefs. Today both men are doing well.

An Important Thing You Can Do

Examine your core beliefs about cancer. Then follow this reframing process:

1. What belief about cancer do you want to change?_____

_____

2. What does holding this belief currently gain you?_____

_____

3. How might you change that belief and view cancer as a positive challenge? (List as many ways as you can.)_____

_____

_____

_____

_____

4. Which of these beliefs and the resulting behaviors would you be willing to try? (Choose at least three.)_____

_____

_____

_____

Reframe cancer by nurturing three responses:

1. Cancer is not so much a threat as it is a challenge.
2. My experience of the illness will be largely determined by the way I think.
3. The way I think is something I can choose. I choose a life of wellness.

#32

EVALUATE
YOUR
SELF-TALK

From the moment we awaken in the morning until we drift off to sleep at night, we experience a constant stream of mental chatter. When we have cancer, our "self-talk" is nearly all negative, filled with fears. It makes for a frightening life experience.

Marion called Cancer Recovery Foundation in a state of panic, her mind reeling out of control. After the first couple of minutes, I began to jot down the opening phrases of her sentences. They give a clear picture of her state of mind:

"The cancer is spreading . . ." "I think my insurance is going to be canceled . . ." "How am I going to pay for this?" "It's all such a burden . . ." "I'm afraid of chemotherapy . . ." "My husband can't deal with this . . ." "I feel so frightened . . ." "Why did this happen to me?" "Where is God when you need him?" "There's nothing I can do."

There is something Marion can do! And you can, too. Believe it or not, we absolutely do choose our every thought. Fear does not overwhelm us without our consent. We may think the same fear-filled thought over and over, out of habit, but we are still responsible for that original choice. Analyze the thoughts you have been holding about cancer. That self-talk is the ancestor of your current experience of illness and of life.

Lou is a woman who has every excuse needed to lead a life of despair. Childhood abuse, a turbulent early marriage, children in trouble, a toxic divorce, a child who ran away, a second husband who died in a work accident, a serious auto accident after which she was disabled for eight months, and then lymphoma. "My mind," explained Lou, "was always filled with thoughts of life being unfair and difficult, a battle."

Then Lou discovered this great truth: Thought is the ancestor of every life experience.

Lou made massive changes. First she came to the profound realization that her troubles were all in her past, over and done. What happened in the past did not automatically predict what would happen in the future. Of primary importance, Lou came to realize that the thoughts and words she chose right here and now were the ones creating her future. Her self-talk set in place her experience, either good or bad.

That was eight years ago. Today Lou is a happy, healthy, and whole person.

An Important Thing You Can Do

Complete this awareness-builder. What positive message can you give to yourself in the following circumstances?

Circumstance: You're angry at the doctor for his arrogance, his impatience with your questions, and the limited amount of time he spends with you.

Positive self-talk: _____

_____

Circumstance: It's 3:00 A.M. and you're wide awake, consumed with thoughts and fears of suffering and self-pity.

*Positive self-talk:*_____

_____

Circumstance: Your energy level is at an all-time low. You are tired and discouraged, questioning if you can take any more.

*Positive self-talk:*_____

_____

   Notice what you are thinking at this moment. Is your self-talk negative or positive? Do you wish for your future to be an extension of these thoughts? Become aware. Choose.

#33

CHOOSE A
DAILY
AFFIRMATION

Affirmations are positive statements of intent and belief. They take the place of the negative mental chatter that may be gripping you. Affirmations serve to "make firm" the positive things about you and your circumstances. They are consciously chosen self-talk.

Affirmations are most powerful when expressed in the present tense. The phrase "I am grateful for life today" is much preferred over a future-tense alternative like "I will show gratitude for my life."

Your words are constantly doing one of two things: building you up or tearing you down; healing or destroying. So affirm positively. You are not so much changing the situation as you are changing your thinking about the situation. Changing your thinking about the disease of cancer may be at the heart of experiencing wellness.

An Important Thing You Can Do

Start now to use the affirmation "I am a picture of wellness," or use some of these:

"I am now receiving unlimited wellness."
"Complete wellness is now mine."
"I love life; this is my moment."
"I am grateful for today!"
"As I sow wellness, I reap wellness."
"I am a 'carrier' of wellness."
"There is nothing in all the world I fear."
"My body is producing miracles."
"I am free from worry. I know peace."
"Wellness is mine, now."
"The Lord is my Shepherd. I shall not want."

#34

MANAGE
YOUR
TOXIC
STRESS

Toxic stress is emotional overload. It is not the stress-causing circumstances themselves, nor is it simply negative emotions. Toxic stress is the *perception* of overload, the overflow of emotions, sometimes expressed but many times suppressed. This perception is experienced in our mind independent of the circumstances. It is under our complete control.

Toxic stress only adds to the physical and mental anguish cancer brings. Stress works at cross-purposes to wellness, putting the mind in a state of confusion, blurring the focused peacefulness needed for healing.

There is something you can do about this perception. It's called the "relaxation response." First named and described by Herbert Benson, M.D., (see section #29) a cardiologist and associate professor of medicine at Harvard Medical School, the relaxation response is a simple, effective, self-healing meditation technique for reducing the detrimental effects of all kinds of stress that we live with every day, particularly the stress associated with a life-threatening illness.

Benson found that the relaxation response is even more effective when one chooses a focus word or phrase that is closely tied to one's spiritual beliefs. The idea is to pick a word or short passage that has meaning for you: a Christian might use *The Lord is my Shepherd* from the Twenty-third Psalm; a Jewish person might choose *shalom*; a nonreligious phrase might be used, such as the word *peace*.

Pick a phrase with significant personal meaning. Dr. Benson calls this the "faith factor" and explains that it can greatly contribute to helping our minds manage stress more effectively.

The quest for daily self-renewal starts with a decision to handle our problems with a sense of equanimity. Eliciting the relaxation response, especially when coupled with the faith factor, results in our minds working for, rather than against, our wellness.

An Important Thing You Can Do

Triggering the relaxation response is simple. Try these steps:

1. Find a quiet place, free from distractions, and sit in a comfortable position.
2. Pick a focus word or short phrase that is deeply rooted in your spiritual beliefs.
3. Close your eyes and relax your muscles, from toe to head, particularly relaxing the shoulder and neck area where most tension is carried.
4. Breathe slowly and naturally. Repeat your focus word silently as you exhale.
5. Assume a passive attitude. When a distracting thought comes to mind, simply dismiss it and return to your focus word.
6. Practice this response for ten to twenty minutes twice a day.

In your Wellness and Recovery Journal, check your daily schedule. Do you have time blocked, twice a day, for stress management? Schedule it. Honor these "appointments."

#35

PRACTICE
VISUALIZATION

An extension of the relaxation process is visualization, also known as mental imagery. This is a valuable tool for helping you reinforce belief in a desired outcome. It is an extension of the relaxation exercises in that it is typically added at or near the end of the meditation period.

The essence of visualization is to create mental pictures of your immune system and of your treatment effectively fighting the cancer. You then visualize the cancer disappearing and your body returning to health. Visualization is that simple, there's no need to make it any more complicated. I urge you to try it.

Consider some of these guidelines: Picture the cancer in either realistic or symbolic terms. For those who require a realistic image, you may want to consult an anatomy text to find pictures of actual cancer cells. Most patients, however, use symbols. I've had people describe their cancer as sand, a lump of clay, and even ice cubes. I saw mine as jelly. The most important criterion for picturing the disease is to think of the cancer as weak and confused. Don't give it power. Your imagery need not be anatomically correct unless you hold a belief that images of correct anatomy are required. What is important is the meaning you give the cancer's imagined symbol; visualize the cancer as weak.

Imagine your treatment as strong and powerful, damaging only the weak cancer cells. Imagine your healthy cells remaining intact. Picture your immune system fighting the cancer. Imagine the weak and damaged cancer cells being naturally flushed out of your body. Picture the cancer shrinking until it is gone. If you are experiencing pain, picture your white blood cells flowing to that area and soothing the pain. Whatever the problem, give your body the command to heal itself, visualizing the process in a way that makes sense to you. End the imagery by seeing yourself well, free of disease, and filled with energy.

How has this benefited you? Most people's fears tend to decrease as the imagery process gives them a greater sense of control. Ongoing research leads us to believe the imagery process has an influence on the body, actually triggering a hormonal and biochemical response to a renewed sense of hope. The resulting changes to the body's chemistry influence immune function, thus assisting the body in maximizing its opportunity to heal.

Visualization is controversial. More than a few health care professionals consider it to be a form of self-deception. "After all," they reason, "I can show you that the tumor has been growing."

I encourage you to consider this response. In your own mind, separate what is happening from what you wish the outcome to be. It is possible, and beneficial, to picture the cancer shrinking even though it may, at this moment, be growing. This is not self-deception. It is self-direction, and is necessary to beginning the pursuit of any life goal. At first, reality will lag behind the vision we have of the desired outcome. But that vision will tend to pull us in the direction we need to go.

How can you make this technique work for you? After evoking the relaxation response, try this:

1. Picture your cancer cells as weak and confused.
2. Create a mental image of your treatment and your immune system overcoming the cancer.
3. Imagine your body's natural processes eliminating the disease from your system.
4. Envision the cancer shrinking until it disappears.
5. Imagine yourself well, filled with vitality for living.

An Important Thing You Can Do

Evoke the relaxation response. Follow it with a visualization exercise. Do so at least daily.

#36

Minimize Treatment Side Effects

Conventional wisdom holds that cancer treatments are ineffective and have drastic side effects. Don't believe it. Conventional wisdom needs to be challenged.

Here's the truth: Cancer treatments are becoming more effective every day. Treatments are also becoming more disease-targeted, affecting fewer healthy cells. Plus several new drugs hold promise for lessening the severity of many of the negative side effects.

Vitally important is the mind's role in combating side effects. In an experiment of a new chemotherapy, part of the group was given saline solution, sterile salt water, as a placebo. Fully 30 percent of this group lost their hair! It is common for patients to experience nausea, not during or after treatment, but on their way to treatment, known as anticipatory nausea. Add to this the legions of examples in which the same treatment results in radically different side effects for different patients, and what do you get? Even allowing for physiological differences, the mind is at work; our beliefs are turned into biological realities.

You and I may perceive our cancer treatments entirely differently. During one of our Cancer Recovery Workshops, I asked Carol, a nursing home administrator, to draw a picture illustrating her body, her breast cancer, and her treatment. A few minutes later she returned with a drawing of a huge devil injecting a charred and smoldering breast with a large syringe of poison. At that same seminar, Rhoda told us that she initially refused both chemotherapy and radiation because she saw them as highly toxic, more threatening than cancer itself. When I asked Rhoda to draw a similar picture, both of her chemotherapy and her radiation therapy, she returned with drawings of chemotherapy as acid eating through a tabletop and radiation therapy as a beam of light that was blinding her vision.

The implications of these images are significant. Negative perceptions of treatment stand in the way of the body's ability to respond favorably. Whenever a patient sees treatment as a friend, a more positive perception starts to work favorably with the treatment. The best way to make treatment a friend is to make certain you "own" the treatment program, knowing that this is what you consider to be the very best treatment at this time.

You can program yourself for the most positive outcome possible by using a type of visualization that athletes have successfully employed in training. After evoking the relaxation response, picture yourself sitting in a chair or lying on a table having your treatment administered. In your mind's eye, see the cancer shrinking. Feel your strength returning. At the end of your imaginary treatment, you feel good and ready to enjoy the gifts of renewed health and greater well-being.

If you do this frequently prior to starting treatment, and especially in the middle of a course of treatment, your body will respond to the actual treatment with maximum capacity and minimal side effects. Like an Olympic athlete, you will be living the event in your mind first. Evidence suggests this helps the body get the message as to how it is expected to respond in the actual situation.

An Important Thing You Can Do

View your treatment as a friend who is there to help you. Take time to "image" your treatment dramatically helping you. Envision yourself as well, free of any treatment side effects, and returning to radiant health.

The steps in this section are basic and fundamental mind/body principles. There's much more to healing with the mind. You may want to continue your training with more reading, attending seminars and workshops, and perhaps personalized instruction. Start with the source list in Chapter #29. Or contact Cancer Recovery Foundation of America, 1-800-238-6479, www.wellness.net.

TOTAL WELLNESS: YOUR NEW LIFE PERSPECTIVE

It is difficult to imagine any benefit coming from the experience of cancer. With the frightening diagnosis, the myriad of treatment decisions, and the need to manage treatment side effects, how could cancer ever be used for good?

Thousands of survivors tell of the real and lasting changes that come directly from their cancer journey. A whole new life may open. This is possible for you, too.

#37

Understand
the
Message
of Illness

When you "reframed" cancer, you began to see illness as more of a challenge than a threat. Now it is time to take this exercise one step further—let's define your unique challenge.

The challenge in illness can be found in its message. In a real sense, the challenge and message of cancer is a call, an opportunity, for personal growth. In this reframe of cancer lies the seed of true healing and lasting wellness.

Could cancer be a message signaling you to make changes in your life? We've already suggested several changes on the physical level—diet, exercise, the lifestyle issues. Might there be more?

Many survivors view cancer as a call for personal transformation. The changes go beyond physical health habits to changes in attitude and self-image. The wise patient uses the experience of cancer as a turning point, a time to replace ineffective and limited ways of coping by substituting healthier, more effective methods of nurturing relationships, developing vocations, and pursuing spiritual growth.

However, as soon as I suggest this position, people cry, "On some level, you're suggesting I subconsciously gave myself cancer!" Not so! We may have participated, but we did not purposely set out to give ourselves a serious illness. Don't read blame, self-sabotage, or guilt into the message of illness. Instead, realize the changes are potential points of power. Understand that if we have participated in our illness, then by definition, we can participate in our wellness.

Many patients who sincerely seek the message of illness often discover a link between their physical, emotional, and even spiritual states of well-being and the onset of their illness. More important, a large number of the survivors whom I have interviewed can trace the beginning of their healing to their decision to change these beliefs and behaviors. They were able to examine the hidden message in illness and choose a response that changed their lives.

I believe that all of us have a personal responsibility to respond to cancer in this manner. Such a response is in your power. Start by asking yourself:

- *What high-stress events or changes happened in the year or two prior to diagnosis?* Become keenly aware of uncontrollable misfortunes. Death of a spouse or child, loss of a job, and financial setbacks are obvious candidates. Also include internal stresses, such as disappointments, major life adjustments, and ongoing conflict in important personal relationships. Most survivors can identify one or more major stresses in their lives prior to the onset of cancer.

- *What was my emotional response to these circumstances?* Did you process your grief over the loss, express your emotions, and finally adopt a hopeful stance; or did you sink into a chronic depressed state? This is a measure of your participation. Don't read blame here. Participation simply refers to how you responded to the circumstances that may have triggered the stress. Might you have put others' needs before your own? Did you give yourself permission to mourn the loss or did you determine you were going to be invincible and show no emotions? Did you permit yourself to seek the support of others during these stresses? How effective was your emotional self-care? Many survivors gain significant insight from a close examination of these questions.

- *How might my reactions to stress and loss be changed?* Are there alternative ways of responding? Could these toxic circumstances and relationships be removed from my life? If not, how can I balance them, honoring my own emotional needs first?

Give yourself permission to define your true needs. This is highly important wellness work. It is perfectly acceptable to find constructive and uplifting ways to meet these needs, regardless of what others may say or think. Give yourself that permission. Understand the message cancer has for you.

An Important Thing You Can Do

Conduct a thorough and unflinching personal inventory. In your Wellness and Recovery Journal, complete this exercise:

1. High-stress event(s) that occurred in the year or two prior to diagnosis or recurrence included_____

_____

_____

2. My three major emotional responses to these high-stress events were_____

_____

_____

3. I could have changed these circumstances by_____

_____

_____

4. I could have changed my emotional response by_____

_____

_____

Complete the inventory and then stop your wellness work for today. Carefully contemplate the implications of the important issues raised in this exercise. You may wish to revise your responses after a time of reflection.

#38

LIVE
THIS
MOMENT

Many people with a diagnosis of cancer needlessly pollute their lives by living in the past or in the future. Instead, I suggest our goal should be to live well with the only time we do have—this very precious present moment.

How many times have you heard yourself say, "If only I hadn't done such and such?" "If only I hadn't smoked." "If only I'd taken better care of myself." "If only . . ." "If only . . ." "If only . . ." We mire ourselves in the regrets of the past and miss the moment we have been given.

At other times we get caught in the fear of the future. "What if such and such happens?" "What if the cancer spreads?" "What if the chemo fails?" "What if . . ." "What if . . ." "What if . . ." Here we miss the present moment because we are consumed with what may happen in the future.

The answer: present-moment living. Live now. Live today. Live this hour. Live this minute to its very fullest. All of our regrets about the past, no matter how sincere, won't change history. All our worries about the future won't add even another minute to our lives. On the contrary, both fears and worries diminish our current minutes by detracting from our ability to enjoy them.

Wellness and happiness are not completely dependent on bodily condition. High-level wellness is possible even with disability. Appreciate the fact that, even with cancer, you have life, here, now. Living each moment fully is the master secret to well-being.

Wellness has everything to do with the quality of our time; it's about this moment. Don't put off living a full life until you are physically "better." Now is the time! This is your moment!

"I was consumed with worry," said Brenda, a non-Hodgkin's lymphoma patient, "not just over my cancer, but about my entire life. My parents were divorced and I worried about my mother's emotional health. My dad traveled a lot and I worried about his airplanes crashing. What about my student loans that still hung over my head, unpaid for several years? Why couldn't I maintain a relationship with a man? Was I just an intractable failure in life? And then my illness, on top of it all."

Corwin was diagnosed with colon cancer at the age of 56. "It [the cancer diagnosis] came two years after my injection molding business failed. All I could think of in those two years was what I should have done differently. If only I had not put so much emphasis on the new product line. Why didn't I see the downturn in the economy? Why did I extend so much credit to our number one customer? I should have announced shorter work weeks or layoffs much sooner. Why didn't I listen to the banker? How am I ever going to get out of debt? If only the family didn't have to suffer. Life is so unfair. I'm ruined."

Brenda and Corwin have a similar problem. Both are absolutely contaminating their present moments. Brenda's worries about the future assure her of enjoying little peace in this moment. Corwin's life is consumed by thoughts of self-judgment that imprison him in the past. Neither is living in the "now." Yet their only chance to capture true wellness is found in the now. What is required is a shift in thinking from what Corwin might have done in the past or what may happen to Brenda in the future, to what each can do right here, right now. What about you? Might similar shifts be required?

Our potential for knowing wellness depends on our ability to understand that the past does not equal the future. Living in the now frees us from an internal bondage that keeps us from following the wellness path.

The past is over. Regrets, remorse, and recrimination cannot touch us unless we allow them to remain in our life. The future cannot harm us unless we create a future based on perceptions of fear, anger, and guilt. The only time that contains the power to change our lives is this present moment.

Just because you have cancer now does not predict, with certainty, that you will have it next year. Understand that truth. You have power in this moment that can change your life. Exercise that power—now!

An Important Thing You Can Do

Each day, relinquish any thoughts or judgments that hold you to the past. Give up any fears that keep you from creating a healthy future. Pick one activity this day, this moment, that brings you pleasure, contentment, and happiness. Do it now! Know that the supply of these moments is limitless, there for the taking if you will only choose to do so. Here, in the present moment, find your wellness.

#39

Take Time to Play

How much time have you allowed yourself for play in the last week? If you answered "None," you are a member of a very large club. That's unfortunate.

Many people react negatively to the idea that we adults need to play. Some believe that grown-ups don't play. Somehow we think that playing is not the mature thing to do. Challenge this thinking. Play is part of the "work" of wellness.

The need to honor our playful nature is very strong. Most of us just repress it. We would do well to give ourselves permission to play, actually scheduling play time in our daily calendars. We must then treat that time carefully, assigning it the same importance and priority as other areas of life, such as work and family.

Sometimes we get fooled into thinking we are playing when we really are not. Ed, who was diagnosed with multiple myeloma, was also a member of a barbershop quartet. He thought his singing was play. Then Ed began to look at his "play" more closely. He soon realized his singing wasn't as much play as it was competition, a pressure to win contests, a pressure he did not need. Ed dropped out of the quartet and substituted kite making, in which the competition was strictly self-imposed. What a valuable lesson!

Analyze your own life. Have you noticed that you're never too tired to play? In fact, if you think you're tired, perhaps that is just the signal that you need more play. Play builds energy reserves; it is a major contributor to wellness.

Consider this list of ten noncompetitive play activities:

1. Stroll on the beach.
2. Fly a kite.
3. Swim.
4. Ride a bike.
5. Draw a picture.
6. Write a poem.
7. Skip around the yard.
8. Sing.
9. Listen to music.
10. Take the scenic route.

An Important Thing You Can Do

Make your own play list and record it in your Wellness and Recovery Journal. Now, stop reading. Put aside this book, right now, and go play for thirty minutes. Go! Have some fun. Do it! We'll continue our wellness work later.

#40

LAUGH
FOR
HEALING
POWER

Norman Cousins made many contributions to our understanding of the mind's role in mobilizing the body's healing processes. But none is so vividly remembered as his emphasis on laughter. In his 1981 book *Anatomy of an Illness,* Cousins called laughter "internal jogging." Since that time, science has confirmed that even something as simple as a laugh or a smile carries with it a positive biochemical response.

The message is clear: Lighten up! It will directly enhance your wellness. Just notice how relaxed you feel after laughing at a good story or watching a funny movie. It's wonderful!

Jack is a New York investment banker, successful, wealthy, the owner of a beautiful home in Westchester County, and the recipient of a metastatic prostate cancer diagnosis. "I thought, my God, I'm going to die. Cancer was the most god-awful threat I had ever faced." Jack received radiation treatment at a Manhattan medical center where he met Delmar, an older gentleman who always had a humorous story to share. Delmar had successfully completed the same treatment for prostate cancer some seven years earlier. Now he volunteered three days a week at the hospital. "My job," said Delmar, "is court jester!"

For most of us, seriousness is seen as an important virtue. We tend to think that laughing or giggling is childish behavior and certainly not appropriate for adults. Jack used to subscribe to this thinking. "After all," he remarked, "investment banking is serous business. You have to be serious to be taken seriously."

Baloney! There is nothing inconsistent about being an adult and including laughter in your life. There is nothing wrong with being ill and pursuing a lighthearted approach to wellness. This need not be some demented form of personal denial. Instead, it can be the opportunity to let the hidden child in you come out once in a while. Get in touch with that exuberant, vibrant part of yourself. Enjoy playing with your own children or grandchildren. Laugh at yourself and your seriousness.

Jack reflected, "Delmar taught me a hell of a lot about living. When I stopped being so damned serious, I started to get well."

An Important Thing You Can Do

Go ahead. Rent that comedy video. Watch your favorite sit-com. Go to the local comedy club or a silly movie. Laugh! Let those positive chemicals and hormones loose. It's healing.

#41

EVALUATE YOUR RELATIONSHIPS

We constantly interact with other people—a husband or wife, a friend or a lover, a child or a relative, a boss, a co-worker, or an employee; the list of our relationships is endless. At times, our lives seem to center entirely on relationships. How we get along with the significant people in our lives seems to determine, to a large extent, the quality of life we have. Furthermore, the absence of relationships can cause much disharmony and deep dissatisfaction. Like it or not, relationships are central to our experience of life and even our experience of illness.

Cancer survivors invest time and energy in relationships that nurture them. Survivors put relationships that are toxic on hold. Patricia shared in a support group meeting what this meant to her. "I had to move out. It was difficult, particularly leaving my two children. But I knew it was what I needed at that time. And I stayed away for nearly three months."

Patricia had married while in college. She went to work to support her husband and his education. Patricia was expecting her first child before her husband graduated from dental school. She never earned her degree, something her husband seemed to hold over her.

"He was always criticizing me," Patricia said. "And I would yell back, trying to defend myself from attack. I'd bring up times when he disappointed me. And he would counter with a litany of my shortcomings. God, it became a vicious cycle. So I got the hell out of there."

Was a marriage gone askew partly responsible for Patricia's cervical cancer? I believe so. Toxic stress lowers our resistance. Patricia's search for love led to an extramarital affair. The guilt became overwhelming, leading to clinical depression. Patricia came to believe the breach in her marriage was linked to her physical problems. After beginning her cancer treatment program, she finally began to look at the relationship with her husband.

Credit Patricia with wanting the relationship to work. With the help of a marriage counselor she was able to better understand her part in the ongoing battles. The counselor helped Patricia recognize her reactions and also helped her select other more appropriate responses to her husband's remarks. Today, Patricia and her husband are working on improving their relationship, and Patricia is cancer-free.

Our relationships with others often reflect the relationship we have with ourselves. Do you experience conflict with a coworker? Look within to understand the inner conflict you may carry. Does a child seem self-willed and impossible? Look within. Do you carry a belief that kids, in general, are willful and impossible?

This internal search is our only real point of influence. When we evaluate relationships, the central task is to look within, discovering the truth: The only way to change another is to change ourselves first.

Do healed relationships always equate with healed bodies? I think the two go together, but I can cite only anecdotal evidence. When we stop punishing ourselves and others for things that happened in the past, we are then free to move on to a life of total wellness, which often supports vast and rapid physical improvement.

An Important Thing You Can Do

Conduct an inventory of the ten most important relationships in your life. Number a page in your Wellness and Recovery Journal from 1 through 10 and record the people's names. Did you realize these were the ten most important people in your life?

Draw a star next to any relationships that need to be put on hold. Are there any that need improvement? Indicate those. What is one thing you could change that would improve each relationship?

Come back to this list weekly. Keep it current. Appreciate how important this work is to your achievement of wellness.

#42

GET
BEYOND
"WHY?"

It's the inevitable question cancer patients ask: "Why did this happen to me?"

The trouble with the "why?" question is that we seldom like the answers we are given. We fight them, not wanting to accept. Some think cancer is a lifestyle issue: "He smoked." That may be true for some but does not stand up to scrutiny for all cancer patients or all smokers. Others say the "why?" is environmental: "We've polluted the planet. We're all getting sick." That may explain some cases, but why is it that other people exposed to the same carcinogens remain perfectly healthy?

Religion tries to answer the "Why me?" question. I've been told by well-meaning clergy that God was using cancer to punish sin, to prevent sin, to correct the patient for his or her eternal profit, to draw unbelievers to God, and to help the patient and family members learn submission. Incredible!

When we ask "why?" we could be looking for someone or something to blame. "Why?" is another way of saying we are helpless and the situation is beyond our control. Some people blame others, some blame circumstances, some blame parents, some blame doctors, some blame the environment, and some blame God. Affixing blame does not help. It only creates helpless victims, something I trust by now you feel you are not.

The road to personal wellness starts when we stop asking "why?" and begin to consider the question, "Toward what end?" or "For what purpose?"—put another way, "How can I make this experience benefit myself, others, and the world?"

An Important Thing You Can Do

In your Wellness and Recovery Journal, start a new page with the heading "How I can make my experience of cancer beneficial." Describe, in writing, how you believe cancer can help you and others physically, emotionally, and spiritually. Continue to add to this list as your insights deepen.

#43

PRACTICE
SELF-DISCIPLINE

Living the well life requires living with values and behaviors that may be radically different from the ones you had before your illness. Some days, the work of wellness may not be the easiest or most convenient to practice. On a cold and rainy morning, it might be easier to stay in bed and forget the exercise. And instead of preparing a high-nutrition lunch, it might seem simpler to use the drive-through window of the nearest fast food restaurant. Our intention to move toward wellness may seem strong, but too often our practices may not reflect that intent.

Wellness self-discipline includes thought and deed, intent and practice. This principle is equally valid whether you are facing a just-baked batch of chocolate-chip cookies, a dark cold morning for exercise, or an unforgivable person. Gentle, wholesome self-discipline is at the core of making wellness real in your life. The issue is not whether we *can* choose wellness. It's whether we *will* choose wellness.

The practice of self-discipline leads to two very powerful life qualities: self-respect and freedom. When your walk matches your talk, when intent and action are one, you have a consistency in your life that is unshakable. You are grounded in a principle-oriented life experience, firm in the knowledge that what you are doing physically, emotionally, and spiritually is in your best interest.

Inner strength and self-respect flow from this position. The discipline to actually act on what is important to you leads to personal freedom; you are no longer bound by the traps of obsession, compulsion, and self-pity. This is personal power at the highest level, a strong and quiet inner assurance that is one of the rewards of the wellness journey.

When I get up in the morning, the first thing I do is pull on my sweats and running shoes. No excuses. I discipline myself to exercise.

Diet was a wellness discipline that challenged me. I loved sweets, especially pastries. Today, I simply do not allow myself to indulge. I deserve better nutrition. Discipline.

Meditation—when do I have time to fit this into a busy schedule? Yet I do, twice each day. Discipline. My times of meditation result in a clearer perspective on the balance of the day that I will not live without.

The same is true for developing a purpose/play balance, nurturing my relationships, and honoring my spiritual needs. Each important area of my life requires a consistent disciplined practice in order for me to know its potential.

"But you're in bondage to your disciplines," protested Manuel, a big burly mechanical engineer with kidney cancer. He was attending one of our workshops in San Antonio. "You're right," I responded, "and so are you." The issue is which habits we will choose in our lives. Choose a positive addiction. Decide to discipline yourself to choose the habits of wellness. The result is self-respect and freedom.

An Important Thing You Can Do

Match your walk with your talk, your actions with your best intentions. Pick one area—perhaps diet or exercise—and make that your focus today. Then choose another area for focus for the next day. And another the next. Feel your self-respect skyrocket. Congratulate yourself. Bask in the personal power and freedom this discipline brings to you.

FOR THE COMMITTED

If you've been following and implementing the steps in this book, you're well on your way to a positive response to cancer. Many cancer survivors go even further, reaching higher levels of well-being in all areas of their lives. "I see it as a gift," says singer and actress Olivia Newton-John about her struggle with breast cancer. "I know it sounds strange. But I don't think I would have grown in the areas that I did without that experience." This can be your experience, too. I urge you to make the commitment.

#44

SEE
LIFE
THROUGH
SPIRITUAL
EYES

What do you see when you look at your life? Do you see a body riddled with disease, dreams hopelessly derailed, a family frightened and in despair?

Or can you see a precious moment, a special instant in space and time where mind and spirit are ill only if you allow it? Can you see the beauty and grace, even the perfection, in your life without coloring those qualities with the pain of cancer?

Peter was a 40-year-old father who developed pancreatic cancer. It was a difficult battle, especially since he wanted so very much to live. His valiant efforts were an inspiration to many people. During one of our telephone sessions, Peter remarked, "I think the spiritual part began to make sense last night. We were at the dinner table, the whole family. And I saw something different. It really stuck with me."

"What do you mean?" I asked.

"Well, before last night, I always saw the obvious at the dinner table: the chicken, the salad, and the mashed potatoes. I'd see my wife, looking tired and worried like she was always running behind schedule. And the kids with a thousand stories of things happening at school. That was what was in front of me. That's what I saw.

"But last night I saw from my heart," continued Peter, struggling to hold back tears. "I looked around that table and saw something quite different. For the first time, I was able to see this precious moment where the minds, bodies, and souls of our family were gathered together to break bread and be nourished. There was so much more there than just the food. There were lives filled with potential for good. We were there to help each other, to love each other, to care for each other."

Peter paused as he relived that special moment in his mind. "Then the children got into an argument with their mother. But instead of driving me up the wall, this conflict was somehow different. Or at least I saw it differently. It seemed to be a natural expression of love toward each other, a way of saying, 'I care.' "

Peter was looking through spiritual eyes. Spiritual eyes allow us to see the value of what is simple and readily available in our lives in spite of the circumstances in which we may find ourselves.

"I awoke from my surgery," said Pontea, "and there in my room was my husband. He was holding our little daughter, propping her up on the hospital bed. And she was squeezing my finger. Her big dark eyes looked at me, and she smiled as she said, 'I love you, Mommy.' It was such a precious moment. Now, since my cancer, I see so much deeper into life."

This level of awareness brings a vastly different experience of illness and of life. Embrace this consciousness. There are miraculous moments in your life right now—every day. You just need to see them.

An Important Thing You Can Do

Tonight, or the next time you are together with family or friends, take a few moments to see life in this new light. Ask yourself, "What do these people really mean to me?" This may contribute more toward your well-being than the most potent medicine.

#45

VALUE
PERSONAL
SPIRITUAL
GROWTH

Too many people equate victory over cancer with a doctor's report that says, "This patient is clinically free of cancer." I understand that desire, I share that desire, and, in fact, my records state exactly that. I wish you the same. But that is not the most important part of the journey through cancer.

Now, read carefully. Consider these next words deeply. For the person who opens his or her mind and spirit, the cancer journey evolves into a spiritual journey. The real triumph over cancer is realized in the nurturing of personal spiritual growth.

Some people say, "I'll settle for a cure. Just get my life back to normal." Don't settle for that! You don't want things to get back to normal. After your experience with cancer, things will never be the same again. You want a new and better life. That life comes in the form of a new spiritual walk.

Cancer has pounded you with a million hammer blows. But you have the last word as to how those blows will shape you. William James, the distinguished psychologist and philosopher, declared that his generation's most important discovery was that human beings, by changing their inner attitudes of mind, could change the outer aspects of their lives.

The hammer blows of cancer can be used to change our inner states of spirit. By making personal spiritual growth our aim, the most important discovery will be to use the experience of cancer to shape us into wonderfully different people. Indeed, cancer can reshape our attitudes, soften our spirits, and transform our lives.

It's personal spiritual growth we seek. Think of personal spiritual growth as a natural extension of your wellness journey. You are going to devote time and energy to getting better. You'll look within to uncover and develop your own practice of gratitude, forgiveness, unconditional love, and more. This is the rewarding call of the work of wellness.

Cynicism has no place here. You cannot climb up the spiritual mountain by thinking downhill thoughts. If you feel that life is filled with despair, that it is gloomy and hopeless, and that spiritual growth is impossible for you, it is because you are gloomy and hopeless. You must change your inner world, which will in turn change your outer world.

Powerful healing awaits you. Associate with men and women who are walking the spiritual path. Your change can be advanced by meeting and mingling with those who have a spiritual vision. Be inspired by our great spiritual ancestors from all the ages.

And pray. Be still and prayerfully listen to the God of your understanding. Don't beg or plead. Pray, "Thy will be done." Then listen. And act. Don't limit God's infinite possibilities by imposing your conditions for wellness. Remember, with God, all things are possible.

An Important Thing You Can Do

In your Wellness and Recovery Journal, record one spiritual quality that you would like to make vivid and real in your life. Start by making a commitment to practice that quality for just one hour. Then extend the time. Keep this as your central goal. Pray and listen for guidance. Opportunities for practice will present themselves every moment of the day. Seize them.

#46

DISCOVER YOUR EMOTIONAL STYLE

What is your dominant style of expressing emotion? Is it suppression, where you constantly restrain yourself from venting real feelings; or overreaction, where you are too exuberant or fly into inappropriate rage; or denial, where you tend to push feelings out of your consciousness?

If you have read this book to this point, you now know that emotions have a central role in wellness. Two emotional styles concern me most: fear that is denied and hostility that is either suppressed or overexpressed. Our goal here is to become a skilled observer of our emotional reactions and learn the ability to choose appropriate responses.

Any and every emotion you feel is perfectly acceptable. We're human; we feel. In a real sense, we are emotionally driven creatures. One moment we're angry, the next moment we're down. We're happy and we laugh. The next moment we're fearful of some loss. I've observed that people tend to repeatedly experience four basic emotions: mad, sad, glad, and e'gad—anger, depression, happiness, and fear. All of them are acceptable.

To experience an emotion, and recognize that any emotion is acceptable, is one level of understanding. But the healthful processing of those emotions is quite another. It's here we typically find trouble.

Health-enhancing emotional processing is summarized by the phrase *review, release, and renew.*

Review the emotion. The most damaging mistake we make in emotional expression is to attach too high a priority on either burying or venting the feeling. Instead, start by observing the emotion. Review it. Understand it. That's half the challenge.

Then release the emotion. Get rid of the anger, the sadness, the fear. It's perfectly acceptable to feel the way you feel. It's your emotion and you need to own it. But then release it in a nonhostile way, without being coy, subtle, or vague. Think or say, "I'm upset but it's only my emotions. It's over and done. My life goes on." Release.

Then renew. Think or say, "I can choose my emotions. My emotions do not choose me." You replace it. Consciously, cognitively, you choose a more productive, more loving, more spiritual emotional response.

This process is so very powerful. For example, my personal emotional challenge is effectively processing anger, one of the most highly charged emotions. My anger is generally short-lived, a negative emotion over a single event. When I'm functioning at my best, I'll review it: "There's my anger. I recognize it. It's starting to boil my water." Then I'll release it: "Please don't say that. I become upset when you act that way." I express it, without malice. I release it.

The trouble comes when I don't renew, when I fail to consciously replace that anger with love, or at least compassion. When I allow anger to continue to control my responses, I am plagued by chronic anger that wears a mask. It appears to be anger but it is actually unresolved hostility— toxic emotions and feelings to which I cling. It's like walking through a field that is filled with landmines. The slightest nudge and an explosion erupts.

One of the demands of living well is to no longer cling to negative emotions. We cling with coping styles of denial, suppression, and overreaction. Not until we review, release, and honestly renew can we become masters of our emotions.

Renewal is actually very simple. For me, it comes when I focus my attention on what actually provoked me. This increased awareness is powerful! If I will just reflect on the event, I will often discover that I perceived the provoker—be it a person, event, or condition—with fear. I was the one who was fearful that my person, property, or pride was under attack.

This is a profound discovery of the highest importance, one that affects us on every level of our lives. It's fear we are dealing with, actually our perception of fear, something that is under our control. Now we can review and release that fear, and verbalize it, "This diagnosis scares me." Or, "Doctor, I am exceedingly uncomfortable with that prognosis."

Then, and only then, can we transcend emotionally. We renew; we consciously choose a more powerful and productive emotion. "I choose to be hopeful—anyway."

Becoming keenly aware of our emotional style, and observing the situations that trigger our emotions, allows us to rethink our fear-based perception that we are under siege. Instead of perceiving fear, we can now understand the situation in the light of hope, or at least compassion. This is a new and miraculous emotional response, one that immediately begins to dissolve resentments and helps in our healing.

Make it your priority to become a keen observer of your own emotional style. Review, release, and renew. It is the secret to emotional well-being.

An Important Thing You Can Do

Become an objective observer over the next week. When an upsetting event occurs, record the event in your Wellness and Recovery Journal. Also record your emotional response based on one of three categories: denial—"I denied that there was any problem"; suppression—"I suppressed my emotions when I really wanted to tell that S.O.B. off"; or overreaction—"I went crazy and overreacted, way out of proportion to the whole event."

Then practice the three Rs: review, release, and renew. You'll become a skilled observer of your own emotional stance toward life. Reactions and emotions that were once automatic will now come under your control. Through it all, you will achieve new levels of well-being.

#47

Make
Forgiveness
a Habit

Do you want to free all your energy to heal? Forgive! Let go!

Forgiveness is wellness work that brings with it huge rewards. Forgiveness links our newfound awareness of the healing dynamics of intimate relationships with our awakened understanding of our emotional style. The promised benefit of this linkage is the peace and serenity we need for healing.

This is a big promise. Forgiveness can deliver.

I believe forgiveness, when it becomes a way of thinking and living, is the single most powerful psychospiritual key to wellness. Forgiveness is a trusted technique by which our thoughts and perceptions are changed, transforming the harmful effects of toxic emotions to the healing reality of compassion, even love. Forgiveness allows us to switch our focus from fear to love; it helps us change what can be changed and allows us to make peace with the rest. This is a requirement of looking at life through spiritual eyes—a profound dimension of healing.

Opportunities to learn and practice the healing lessons of forgiveness are everywhere. The teachers of forgiveness come disguised as people, most often individuals who antagonize us, the ones whom we can't stand to be around.

We effectively teach ourselves the lessons of forgiveness when we hold ourselves accountable to be self-forgiving. Let's be honest; we hold many resentments against ourselves; we don't let go easily. In the quiet moments we judge ourselves harshly, "I'm so stupid. I'm fat. I'm ugly." The list is without end. Now, like never before, this is the moment to release that self-condemnation. The only way is through self-forgiveness.

Let go. I observe so many cancer patients carrying self-concepts of unworthiness. This is a false and deadly belief. Yes, we may have done something undesirable, but that is our behavior and does not equate with being an unworthy person. Release those feelings of unworthiness.

There's more. Our perceptions of others can also create a battleground of emotional turmoil. It is so easy to judge others. Judgmental behavior tears at the fabric of relationships and kindles the fires of resentment. Cancer is, among other things, an opportunity to learn and practice the difference between acceptance and approval, to transcend judgment.

Forgiveness is the answer. All of us have imperfect natures. All of us exhibit behaviors that don't match our potential. Forgiveness allows us to accept imperfection without having to approve of it. Have you noticed? Not everything in life meets your expectations. But we can find peace through acceptance. Forgiving ourselves and others is at the heart of practicing acceptance.

Let's begin to make the practice of forgiveness a habit. Forgiveness is experienced on two levels. The first is the most obvious. There is an event: Someone is wronged or we perceive an attack. That behavior needs to be forgiven. When we can say, "I forgive myself for _____," or "I forgive _____ (another) for _____," then we have embarked upon the forgiveness journey.

The second level of forgiveness changes our perception of what happened. Yes, an event occurred. But the real problem starts when we begin to judge what happened, when we label ourselves or the other person as bad, hurtful, mean, stupid, or with some other less-than-kind attribute. We perceived the event as unfavorable; the event didn't meet our approval. We judge, even condemn, the people involved.

The alternative? Acceptance. Accept ourselves. Accept others. Accept that events happen. Accept that life is often far from our glittering ideals. Forgive and accept. This is a far better way to live.

People who are, or believe themselves to be near death often come to the realization that forgiveness heals. Feuds, differences, and deep hurts suddenly seem less important at this time. I can understand. I had to learn this lesson myself. Literally thousands of patients share similar stories.

Marilyn, in the middle of a battle with ovarian cancer, felt terribly ill at ease when her mother and father visited. Marilyn and her mother would make noble efforts to get along with each other, but they seldom fully succeeded. Old patterns of attack and defense were constantly cropping up between them. Child care, cooking, homemaking, religion—the particulars didn't seem to matter. Her mother wanted a more conservative daughter. Marilyn wanted a more enlightened mother.

"It was driving me crazy," said Marilyn. "During her last visit, I was ready to throw her out. But then it occurred to me, God isn't looking at my mother and thinking, 'Mildred is such a bitch.' How could I pretend to want to get along with my mother if I was so consumed by my judgment of her errors? I had to practice acceptance and get off my fixation with approval.

"So I said to myself, 'I'll try this for an afternoon. I'll focus on acceptance and give up approval.' From that moment, the situation and the relationship started to shift. As I was more accepting of her, she became more accepting of me. We're a long way from best buddies," conceded Marilyn, "but there is a growing bond between us."

The amazing payoff of forgiveness is that so many people do get well after extending forgiveness! Lives are certainly made better; many are made longer. But it strikes me that if one is willing to forgive during the last moments of life, why not do it earlier? Like right now?

How often do we need to forgive? Always. Don't drag the memories of past hurts and mistakes into your present moments. Nothing from the past is important enough to allow it to pollute our present. Forgive. Let go of judgment. Become a shining example of compassion. You deserve it. You'll change your life—forever!

An Important Thing You Can Do

Choose one hurt or mistake and forgive everyone concerned with it. Say out loud, "(Name), I totally and completely forgive you." Mean it. Now feel the warmth of forgiveness. It's called freedom—and wellness! Choose to forgive one person each day.

#48

EXUDE
GRATITUDE

What is the least-healthy spiritual habit, the one that causes disease of every kind? It's ingratitude—the lack of thankfulness, our inadequate appreciation for all the blessings we enjoy.

Have you expressed your thankfulness today? We all have so many blessings to appreciate every day of our lives. But most of us overlook them. The conscious practice of being grateful is central to the healing process.

Even with cancer, even in the middle of difficult treatment, even in your darkest and most fearful hours, be thankful for all you do have. For life, for love, for family, for friends, for the awesome beauty of nature, for the presence of God, for all these things and more, be thankful.

Thousands of survivors are convinced that there is a physiological correlative to gratitude; their bodies respond.

If you wish to cultivate a deeper attitude of gratitude, I suggest you begin to see yourself as a guest who is only visiting here on earth. All that you have is not really yours; it is a gracious gift from your host. You are privileged to enjoy the gifts of friends and family, home and transportation, food and recreation, vocation and service, during your stay. Even your health, no matter what the state, is another of those gifts.

Jill lay near death in a small rural Nebraska hospital after being told she was "filled" with cancer and that it was inoperable. Mired in despair and self-pity, she could see nothing for which she could be thankful. "I was divorced, my two children were grown and lived in different parts of the country. I hated my dead-end job. My life seemed miserable.

"But one night I looked out of my hospital window to see a deep dark sky that was filled with stars. I shut off all the lights in my room and just gazed at that sky for what must have been hours. I started to ask a lot of questions: 'What is this huge universe about? What is my place in it? Why am I sick?' I can't say I got a lot of answers. But I did get a different perspective.

"I became thankful," continued Jill, "grateful just for being a part of this huge and wonderful world. I realized that in my fifty-plus years, I had been able to experience so much. The marvel of giving birth to two other lives—what a miracle! The beauty of the country, where I feel such strong roots; I was so grateful to live here rather than in a city. The deep friendship I had with my sister—I was so thankful for her love. That night at the window changed my whole perspective on my problems."

Like Jill, we too can capture true wellness when we choose gratitude. But so many roadblocks on the cancer journey seem to detour us, to mire us in ruts of ingratitude and self-pity. We're so busy with appointments and treatments, discomfort and despair, fear and pain, some moments even suffering, that we lose our perspective. We tend to look at the cancer journey as a long and twisted path, filled with potholes. There seems to be nothing for which we can be thankful. This is faulty and self-destructive thinking.

Gratitude transforms the very experience of illness and of life. Gratitude is one component of viewing the world with spiritual eyes. I implore you, see beyond the day-to-day experiences that seem so all-consuming. Treasure the wonder of life. Become aware of your "guest status" in this brief moment in time and space. Be thankful. It heals.

An Important Thing You Can Do

It's time for another page in your Wellness and Recovery Journal. Label it, "Today I am thankful for:" You may want to divide the page into three columns: People, Places, and Things. Be thankful for all the gifts. Express your gratitude.

#49

PRACTICE UNCONDITIONAL LOVING

Loving heals. Even though there may be times when we are lost in the abyss of our physical maladies or buried in the agony of our emotional awfulizing, with each moment comes a new opportunity to choose loving. This is a decision that truly heals.

Loving without conditions is an intentional choice that determines what is coming *through* us rather than what is coming *to* us. The choice to love means we don't have to wait for the medical test results, the doctor's assurances, the elusive remission, or the hoped-for cure. We can choose to love now, this moment. And the next moment. And the next. We always have this power of choice, regardless of the circumstances.

I prefer the word *loving* over *love*. It denotes the action necessary to bring the idea of love to life. Love is not loving until it is released, until it is intentionally given.

Consider this perspective. The crippling fears surrounding cancer are actually the absence of love. The fear is like darkness that is merely the absence of light. You don't solve a problem of darkness by yelling at it or trying to strike at it. If you want to get rid of the darkness, you turn on a light.

So it is with fear. You don't fight it. You replace fear with loving.

This is a profound and radical call, not some live-with-loving-feelings suggestion. Loving is more than a thin veneer. Loving is an act of heroism and courage of the highest order. You should not seek or even expect accolades. Unconditional loving is not a decision surrounded by pomp and circumstance. Most often it has to do with small choices. "How do I choose to respond to this person?" "How might I focus on the positive?" "How would exercising nurture my total well-being?" "How can I best help another person?" "How can I best love myself?"

By most standards, the conditions and circumstances of cancer do not inspire loving. Taken by themselves, the conditions may elicit despair; the cancer journey has many such moments. But we can take the loving action anyway! Invariably, the result is a renewed sense of hope that results in a strong biochemical "live" signal to body, mind, and spirit.

Loving starts with self-loving. You can hope to know wellness only from a position of personal emotional and spiritual strength. Self-loving is the wellspring of this vital force. Affirm your great value; cancer does not detract from your self-worth. Self-loving is the root of recovery for thousands of patients.

Does loving seem too difficult a task? Does your mind say that you can never be at peace until the cancer is gone? Do you feel that a total and complete physical cure is the only acceptable answer? Does it seem impossible to love with the sword of cancer balancing precariously over your head?

Love anyway. For if you love, you will be healed.

Loving is the first and last word in healing, the great balm that quiets distress, the only real "magic bullet" against cancer, and the strongest vaccine to combat malignancy.

Our greatest enemy is not disease but despair. Unconditional loving is the healer.

An Important Thing You Can Do

It is decision time. Decide to practice unconditional loving for the next hour. And the next hour, and the next. You will know healing—something far greater than a cure.

#50

SHARE
THIS
HOPE

Now that you've invested time reading this book and following at least some of the steps, you're aware that there is much you can do to improve your well-being. Your choices and actions really do make an enormous difference. In partnership with your medical team, you are on the pathway to healing.

But most people don't know these powerful truths. Or if they do, they have only a vague acquaintance with the strategies, not a working knowledge. They deserve more.

Share this hope with others who have been diagnosed with cancer. Discuss these ideas. Encourage one another. Make it your new priority to walk the path of wellness with someone else. This has the cumulative effect of helping yourself while helping another.

Please contact us. We have a free newsletter for you, plus a variety of helpful wellness resources. You have a caring partner in your journey.

The Cancer Recovery Foundation of America
P.O. Box 238, Hershey, PA 17033
(800) 238-6479 / www.wellness.net

EPILOGUE:
YOU
HAVE
A FUTURE

While cancer is certainly a serious illness, anyone who has fought the battle knows that it is as much a psychological and spiritual battle as a physical one. They also know what a meaningful contribution the mind and spirit can make.

Tap deeply into the mental and spiritual assets with which you have been endowed. Use illness as an opportunity for personal growth. That may seem beyond the scope of your current thinking. But believe that it can be accomplished. Illness has been the pathway for millions of people to discover an even better life than they ever dreamed possible. Illness can be your wakeup call, a chance to experience the life you may have been forced to put on hold.

No matter how much time you think you may have to live, make the decision to live today—fully! Make the profound choices to forgive and to love. This leads to a better life and, as thousands of us believe, a longer life as well.

Let this illness be your new beginning. Choose to be well this moment. A hopeful, happy future can be yours. Choose it now. It's truly the essential thing you can do when the doctor says, "It's cancer."

APPENDIX A:
IF CHEMOTHERAPY
IS RECOMMENDED

If you sense I am skeptical about chemotherapy, you are correct. I want you to know of my belief and balance it with your own convictions as you make your treatment choice.

The guiding dictum of the Hippocratic Oath is "First, do no harm." Chemotherapy does not adhere to this principle. Simply put, the goal of chemotherapy is to harm cancer cells by poisoning them in order to disrupt their ability to grow and multiply. Sometimes, in some types of cancers, it works. However, in the process, your host defense system is typically harmed, and at high doses, often irreparably compromised. Tumors that initially respond to treatment frequently develop a resistance to these toxic drugs. While a tumor may respond a second time, the response is often at a lower level of effectiveness. In the meantime, quality of life often suffers. Worse, the body may be weakened to a point where less-invasive alternatives have little chance to effectively rebuild immune function, extend life, or yield quality-of-life gains.

Clearly, chemotherapy does have its place. Good science

shows chemotherapy to be efficacious in producing a cure in most cases of Hodgkin's disease, acute lymphocytic leukemia, and testicular cancer. Chemotherapy is also effective in a handful of relatively rare, mainly chilchood cancers, including Burkitt's lymphoma, lymphosarcoma, and choriocarcinoma. With surgery and/or radiation, chemotherapy plays a role in the successful treatment of Wilms' tumor, Ewing's sarcoma, rhabdomyosarcoma, and retinoblastoma.

Research shows chemotherapy seems to be effective in extending life in many cases of ovarian cancer. In small-cell lung cancer, chemotherapy seems to effect a life extension of several months. However, in both of these cases, chemotherapy by itself does not seem to effect a cure and quality of life typically suffers.

At best, the evidence is much less clear in the now-common practice of employing chemotherapy as an adjunctive treatment in breast cancer. In premenopausal women, there may be a small statistical advantage, approximately a 4 percentage point gain, in survival rates for those who take chemotherapy. But this gain must be balanced with the very real potential for collateral damage caused by the same chemotherapy, the most common being the impairment of heart, liver, kidney, and pancreatic functions. In other words, while the chemotherapy seems to marginally reduce the risk of the breast cancer spreading, it concurrently increases the risk of other potentially serious health problems.

For postmenopausal women with breast cancer, a statistically stronger case can be made for tamoxifen. However, tamoxifen has been linked with increased incidence of endometrial cancer, uterine cancer, liver cancer, damage to the eyes, and blood clots that may have led to stroke and coronary thrombosis in clinical trial participants. Tamoxifen is perhaps best suited to a narrow group of high-risk breast cancer patients who take the drug in order to reduce the risk of cancer in the second breast.

Chemotherapy's one other area of limited demonstrated success is colon cancer. There still is no conclusive evidence of its effectiveness except after lymph node involvement. Yet even though the clinical evidence is unclear, current conventional

American practice says try chemotherapy in virtually all cases of colon cancer.

In my opinion, what is happening is that oncologists in the United States are administering chemotherapy to more patients, across a wider spectrum of malignant disease, in the hope that it may show results. The cancer community has tended to extrapolate their narrow successes and consider nearly all cancer patients, especially those with metastatic or recurrent disease, as candidates for chemotherapy. This is the "why" behind my reservations and this urgent warning to understand clearly what chemotherapy will and will not accomplish.

The fact is, in the treatment for types of cancers beyond those mentioned above, conclusive proof of chemotherapy's effectiveness in the form of large randomized clinical trials is simply nonexistent. Even in those cancers where tumor response has been demonstrated, current chemotherapy regimens alone fail to consistently deliver the outcomes of curing the patient, prolonging life, or improving quality of life. It is the multifaceted integrated approach emphasized throughout this book that is crucial to understand and implement.

Special Note to Patients Who Choose Chemotherapy

Having explained my reservations, I want to state that chemotherapy may be right for you. One important correlation with any treatment's success is the belief the patient brings to the process. It is understandable that many people choose chemotherapy based on belief in tumor response; it makes theoretical sense to reduce the tumor burden and then begin to systematically rebuild one's immune function. Add to this the fact that the medical community widely accepts and supports chemotherapy, that the insurance industry regularly reimburses for its administration, and that cancer research dollars are heavily invested in this modality, and this choice of treatment comes with a great deal of built-in support. With all that evidence, it's believable.

If you do choose this therapy, I urge you to use extreme caution in approving high-dose chemotherapy. Results of five breast cancer studies on the use of high-dose chemotherapy with autologous bone-marrow or stem-cell transplant found no conclusive benefit from the more aggressive therapy. Specifically, data in four of the five studies show no significant difference in survival of patients receiving the high-dose regimen as compared with those receiving lower-dose chemotherapy without transplants. This data directly challenges earlier studies and widely held assumptions that indicated increased survival rates.

Is there a middle ground? One chemotherapy strategy to consider is fractionated or smaller dosages infused over an extended period of time. The highly toxic effects are typically minimized because the lower or diluted dose does not create dangerous systemic toxicity. In fact, evidence exists that low-dose chemotherapy appears to offer the added benefit of actually stimulating the immune system. Although many conventionally trained oncologists will dismiss the effectiveness, I predict this homeopathic "less-is-more" approach will become as widely accepted in American chemotherapy circles as it now is in other countries.

If you choose to undergo chemotherapy or have already had chemotherapy, study carefully this book's chapters #22, "Follow These 'Eat-Smart' Guidelines," and #25, "Determine Your Vitamin, Mineral, and Herbal Supplements." Start strengthening and rebuilding your immune system now. If you have a recurrence, I suggest you fully explore your immunotherapy options.

APPENDIX B:
NONTOXIC AND LESS TOXIC CANCER TREATMENTS

The explosion of public interest in alternative cancer therapies makes this appendix appropriate to the revised edition of *Cancer: 50 Essential Things to Do*. I support patient freedom of choice in medical care. My concern is that these nonconventional choices be made with full knowledge of the expected outcomes, the same standards which we must more rigorously apply to conventionally accepted treatments.

Two resources stand out for your evaluation of complementary and alternative treatment options. The book:

Moss, Ralph. *Cancer Therapy: The Independent Consumer's Guide to Non-Toxic Treatment & Prevention.* New York: Equinox Press, 1992, 1997.

The definitive website for research on alternative treatments is the Center for Alternative Medicine Research in Cancer. Run by the University of Texas, it is funded by the Office of Alternative Medicine at the National Institutes of Health and represents the first objective and dispassionate evaluation of some of the most controversial cancer treatments. Open the site at:

www.sph.uth.tmc.edu/utcam

Spend quality time with both of these resources prior to making decisions on nontraditional treatments. Remember our findings: The vast majority of cancer survivors integrate conventional treatment with a variety of complementary and alternative techniques. At our current level of understanding cancer treatment, integration remains the strategy of choice.

APPENDIX C:
A CANCER
PATIENTS'
BILL OF
RIGHTS

Medical freedom of choice is fundamental to a free society. A cancer patient's effort to take responsibility for those choices must begin immediately upon diagnosis. That is often a time when the patient is in shock. It is also a time when the cancer patient who intends to survive must mobilize the will to live.

Unfortunately, too many doctors routinely impose traditional cancer treatment approaches without giving the patient the benefits of understanding his or her full course of options. In part, the doctors do so because they view themselves as lifesavers. And in practice, many patients seek just that, someone who has all the answers and will help them recover with minimal effort and discomfort.

The United States Senate has before it a proposed Patients' Bill of Rights. This legislation focuses mainly on insuring access to medical care. The bill is considered to be pro-consumer in that it guarantees patients' rights when dealing with health insurance companies, health maintenance organizations (HMOs), and other managed care programs.

The clear emphasis of the proposed bill is ensuring guaranteed access to conventional medical solutions. However, with conventional cancer therapies, the risk of overtreatment is at least as great as the risk of undertreatment. Conventional cancer treatment modalities—surgery, radiation, and chemotherapy—are both highly invasive and toxic. They may, and often do, cause serious and lasting physical impairment, frequently without effecting a cure.

I believe the patient right that must be guaranteed is full information regarding all treatment options, including less-invasive and less-toxic alternatives. In addition to assured access to emergency care, specialty care, continuity of care, clinical trials, and choice of providers, I wish to propose a special Cancer Patients' Bill of Rights and Responsibilities that will promote full freedom of medical choice and thus maximize recovery potential.

Cancer patients in the United States of America shall:

1. Have the right to a full and complete understanding of their diagnosis. Basic to making informed treatment choices is to know what they are fighting.
2. Have the right to a copy of their medical records.
3. Have the right to a second, third, or fourth medical opinion.
4. Have the right to demand answers to questions in understandable language.
5. Have the right to ask for proof of effectiveness of the treatment being offered. They shall have the further right to evaluate this evidence in terms of actual cure, increased survival time, and improved quality of life, not just tumor response.
6. Have the right, provided they are mentally competent adults, to accept or refuse any cancer treatment. Furthermore, they shall have the right to continue with any treatment, even if they or their doctors believe the chances are minimal that the treatment will be helpful. They shall also have the right to discontinue any cancer therapy.

7. Have the right to seek entry into an experimental protocol sponsored by the National Cancer Institute or another similar organization, even though such programs may not be reimbursed by health insurance carriers or endorsed by their oncologists.

8. Have the right to choose complementary treatments including special diets and nutritional supplements.

9. Have the right to choose alternative cancer therapies and work with an alternative practitioner, even though such programs may not be reimbursed by health insurance carriers or endorsed by the government.

10. Have the right to work with loved ones and health care providers to maximize function and comfort, and prepare for eventual death by living well in the moment.

11. Have the right to reject any health care provider's estimate of how long they may have to live.

12. Have the right to integrate emotional resources, religious or spiritual beliefs and practices into their treatment and recovery program.

In short, I propose and affirm the fundamental right to choose the cancer treatment program which enjoys one's greatest confidence, even if that means refusing all treatment. Patients do not have to be seen as "reasonable" or live up to anyone else's expectations, including a doctor's.

Once again, the risks of overtreatment are at least as great as the risks of undertreatment. For your own body, mind, and spirit, you alone are responsible and autonomous.

SURVEY ON
CANCER
AND
RECOVERY

Your help is needed. If you are eighteen years of age or older, please take a few moments to answer the following questions. Please use a separate sheet of paper. Including your name and address is optional.

The purpose of this survey is to learn in greater depth how people respond to cancer. Your experiences could be of significant help to others who are confronting the illness.

The combined responses of this questionnaire will be published in a variety of forms. However, no respondent will be identified by name without prior written permission. Please indicate if you are willing to be identified. All answers to the questions are voluntary. If you do not want to answer a question, feel free to skip it and go on to the next one.

1. Describe your type of cancer, the month and year of initial diagnosis and recurrence, if applicable, and the recommended treatment(s). Did you obtain a second opinion? Were you treated by a board-certified oncologist?

2. What was the most difficult part, physically, emotionally, and spiritually? Be specific. Include as many details as possible.

3. How did your cancer affect your family, including spouse, children, and/or parents? Who was the most helpful? Least helpful? Why?

4. How has cancer affected your faith? How has your faith impacted your cancer?

5. In addition to medical doctors, have you sought professional help from a psychologist, a member of the clergy, and/or others? Please rate the effectiveness of the help you received from each professional.

6. Did you use nontraditional treatment(s)? Which ones? Please comment on your experiences and/or impressions.

7. Have you attended a cancer support group? If yes, who was the sponsor? How often do you attend? How would you rate the effectiveness of the help?

8. Has cancer challenged the fundamental values by which you live your life? If so, in what ways?

9. What advice do you have for someone who is confronting a cancer diagnosis?

10. Was this book helpful to you? What was most helpful? Least helpful?

Please mail your response to this survey to:

Survey on Cancer and Recovery
The Cancer Recovery Foundation of America
P.O. Box 238
Hershey, PA 17033
e-mail: www.wellness.net

Thank you for sharing.

ABOUT
THE
AUTHOR

Greg Anderson was diagnosed with metastasized lung cancer in 1984. He was given only 30 days to live. Refusing to accept the hopelessness of this prognosis, he went searching for people who had lived although their doctors had told them they were "supposed" to die. His findings, from interviews with over 15,000 cancer survivors, form the strategies and action points of this powerful and hope-filled book.

In 1985 Greg started the Cancer Conquerors Foundation, the predecessor of Cancer Recovery Foundation of America. This organization provides training and support for implementing body-mind-spirit wellness strategies. Services include seminars, workshops, support groups, audiovisual programs, self-assessment tools, and a free newsletter, "Creating Wellness."

The Anderson family lives in Central Pennsylvania. Prior to his illness, Greg was vice-president and executive director of the Robert Schuller Institute, located at the Crystal Cathedral in Garden Grove, California. He is the author of six additional books, including *Healing Wisdom, The Cancer Conqueror, Journeys with the Cancer Conqueror,* and *The 22 (Non-negotiable) Laws of Well-ness.* Today he travels extensively to speak and conduct workshops, sharing his experience and techniques. He may be contacted at Cancer Recovery Foundation of America, P.O. Box 238, Hershey, PA 17033, U.S.A.; (800) 238-6479; greg@well ness.net.